Ethics in Nursing

DATE DUE

To
Mary Nielsen and Gary Davies
whose deep caring has enabled me to care,
I dedicate this book.

Ethics in Nursing

The caring relationship

Second edition

Verena Tschudin, BSc(Hons), RGN, RM, Dip.Couns

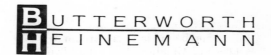

Butterworth-Heinemann Ltd
Linacre House, Jordan Hill, Oxford OX2 8DP

✒ PART OF REED INTERNATIONAL BOOKS

OXFORD   LONDON   BOSTON
MUNICH   NEW DELHI   SINGAPORE   SYDNEY
TOKYO   TORONTO   WELLINGTON

First published 1986
Reprinted 1989, 1990
Second edition 1992
Reprinted 1992

British Library Cataloguing in Publication Data
Tschudin, Verena.
    Ethics in nursing: The caring relationship – 2nd ed.
    I. Title
    174.2

ISBN 0 7506 0346 1

Library of Congress Cataloging in Publication Data
Tschudin, Verena.
    Ethics in nursing : the caring relationship / Verena
    Tschudin – 2nd ed.
    p.   cm.
    Includes bibliographical references and index.
    ISBN 0 7506 0346 1
    1. Nursing ethics.   I. Title.
    RT85.T73   1992
    174'.2–dc20   91–29734
                                                          CIP

Printed and bound in Great Britain by
Biddles Ltd, Guildford and King's Lynn

Contents

Preface to the second edition   vii

1   Caring: a basis for ethics   1

2   The caring relationship   17

3   Values and value-statements   28

4   Ethical theories   46

5   Codes and declarations   64

6   Responsibilities and rights   74

7   Making ethical decisions   82

8   Ethical issues in nursing   93

9   Ethical dilemmas   131

10   Ethics and the future   150

Postscript   164

References   165

Index   173

Preface to the second edition

Sometimes ethics seems like a river in the landscape of life. It flows on in the course carved out, but it constantly changes its aspects. It flows through uplands and lowlands, through open spaces and through gorges, sometimes quietly, sometimes forcefully.

Like a river, ethics is a necessary part of life. We can go over it or tunnel under it, take a boat across it or swim through it. Some people just sit on the edge, watching it. We can try to avoid ethics, or not see it, feel above it, or be immersed in it; but we cannot avoid it. Like the river, it is there, giving life and taking from it.

Writing the second edition of this book was at times like a baptism by a total immersion in the river which fascinates and challenges me. Sometimes I feel I tried to build dams across it, and at other times I saw my own image reflected. Whatever I try to do to, and with, this river, it certainly does a lot to, and with, me!

Because so much has changed in the field of ethics since the first edition was published, this second edition is more like a new book that simply a revision. Not only has material been updated, but aspects which seem relevant to the present have been added and others dropped. The theme of an ethic of caring has been strengthened and followed through more vigorously.

An ethic of caring is not something clearcut, like some theory might be. On the contrary, it is something which disturbs patterns, asks awkward questions, and puts emphasis on aspects which are not easily dealt with. This may mean that some people find it uncomfortable. Our age is geared towards competition and to acquiring more of everything: knowledge, money, speed, goods and health. An ethic of caring does not deny any of this, but may look at it from the point of view of the persons concerned, in this instance the care-receiver and the care-giver. This gives it a dimension which may not always be familiar to the textbooks. But it will be familiar to those concerned, because it involves their humanity.

My hope is that this second edition will be not only a help towards ethical thinking and practice for nurses and colleagues, but also a stimulant to look for what is human, and therefore joyous and beautiful.

Particular thanks go to all those people who in discussion and lectures have stimulated me to think more clearly and question more penetratingly, and those who told of their difficult situations and asked for help with them. A special thank you to Susan Devlin, Senior Medical Editor of Butterworth-Heinemann, for seeing this edition painlessly through its various stages. An affectionate thank you goes to Margaret Wellings for typing yet another manuscript from scrap paper, while a word processor is waiting idle in the cupboard.

Verena Tschudin
London, 1991

Caring: a basis for ethics

The uniqueness of caring

Everybody cares these days. The bank cares. The waste-disposal people care. This garage mechanic cares more and that hand-cream cares most of all. Since everybody and everything cares, some would say, the idea of caring has become cheap. Nothing is special about it any more. This may be true to some extent; caring is not unique *to* nursing, but it is still unique *in* nursing.

Most books on ethics start with concepts such as morality, or principles, or values. Issues such as emotions, affection, experience and relationships are then treated as subject to these time-honoured ways of seeing the world.

Nursing, however, is a practical, hands-on job, where experience, emotion, affection and relationships make up the bulk of everyday work. It seems reasonably, therefore, to start a book on ethics in nursing from that point of view.

Caring is about people. It is done with people, for people, to people and as people. It is this last aspect which makes caring unique: people relate to people; one person relates to another person.

Caring

In order to understand the uniqueness of caring in nursing, a few general ideas about caring may help.

In a small book simply entitled *On Caring* Milton Mayeroff (1972) lists eight 'major ingredients' as necessary for caring.

Knowledge

In caring we need to know many things: who the other is, what his needs are and what helps him. We also need to know ourselves and our strengths and limitations. We know some things explicitly and others implicitly. 'One important reason, perhaps, for our failure to realize how much knowing there is in caring is our habit sometimes of restricting knowledge arbitrarily to what can be verbalized.' Knowledge is conveyed both verbally and non-verbally.

Alternating rhythms

We move between past experience and the present situation, between narrow and wide frameworks, between attention to detail and attention to the whole. Both are necessary – both are part of caring.

Patience

We do not only wait passively for something to happen, we give our full attention. But like an idea, or the growth of a child, the growth of a person into full potential may take time. When we care we have patience with the person and go at his pace.

Honesty

This is a positive, often active, confrontation between ourselves and the other. We need to see the other as he or she is, not as we would like him or her to be.

Trust

This involves an appreciation of the other, of his or her independent existence. When we care too much, when we 'overprotect' the other, then we are not mutually trusting. But trusting also means that we have confidence in our ability to help. We must trust ourselves and our instincts.

Humility

When we are open to each person and situation, then each relationship is unique. We cannot simply do what we did in the last case; we have to learn all the time. This learning means constant restarting. Humility also sees others as existing for themselves, and not simply to satisfy our needs. Caring also teaches us our true limitations and strengths. We accept both with humility.

Hope

Hope is not wishful thinking, but an expression of the fullness of the present, a present alive with a sense of the possible. The process of caring is possible only because hope is always present.

Courage

In caring, in growing, we go into the unknown. Courage makes risk-taking possible. But courage is not blind. It is informed by knowledge of the past and by trust in our own and the other's ability to grow.

Caring can only be experienced, and the quality of that experience is what matters. These ingredients help to shape the quality of caring in general.

The 'Five Cs' of caring

The Canadian nurse-philosopher M. Simone Roach (1987) has also established a set of aspects of caring. These are related particularly to nursing, but grow out of her general statement that 'Caring is the human mode of being'. Care is the basic element of being a person. When we do not care, we lose our 'being', and caring is the way back into 'being'.

The old division had it that doctors cure and nurses care. But Nouwen (1987) points out that 'care is the basis and precondition of all cure', and as a doctor once said, caring was done much before curing was done.

Caring embodies certain qualities and specific characteristics. Roach has found that these all start with the letter 'C': compassion, competence, confidence, conscience and commitment.

Compassion

> Compassion may be defined as a way of living born out of
> an awareness of one's relationship to all living creatures.

The word compassion has an old-fashioned ring to it. The
outmoded expression 'bowels of compassion' may point to the
fact that compassion is often the response of a gut feeling to a
situation of great need or 'passion'. Compassion is a specific act
in response to a specific need.

Nouwen (1982) writes that:

> Compassion asks us to go where it hurts, to enter into places
> of pain, to share in brokenness, fear, confusion and anguish.
> Compassion challenges us to cry out with those in misery,
> mourn with those who are lonely, to weep with those in
> tears. Compassion requires us to be weak with the weak,
> vulnerable with the vulnerable, and powerless with the
> powerless. Compassion means full immersion in the condition
> of being human.

Compassion is more than simple kindness. It is also more than
caring; we *can* care without having compassion. Compassion is
something both decisive and incisive.

> The wounded surgeon plies the steel
> that questions the distempered part;
> Beneath the bleeding hands we feel
> the sharp compassion of the healer's art
> Resolving the enigma of the fever chart (Eliot, 1944)

There is in this poem the implication that compassion only comes
after an experience of being wounded onself. When we have been
'bleeding' ourselves, and have experienced compassion shown us,
then we can – out of that experience – in turn be healers.
Compassion is something that we only know by experience. We
cannot learn how to have or apply it. We cannot study it; no
programme in sensitivity will give it to us. We can only be
compassionate because compassion has been shown towards us.

Churchill (1977) believes that in nursing:

> Compassion is the groundwork, competence the superstructure. Usually in thinking of health professionals, we reverse this; we try to train a competent professional, and tack on compassion as a finishing touch – icing on the cake, a highly desirable frill. To me this bespeaks a root poverty of our ability to really see *what* health professionals do, and *how deeply* they generally affect the lives of those they serve.

Competence and competitiveness are closely linked. Nouwen (1982) believes that nowadays competition, not compassion, is our main motivation in life. We judge people by what they *do*, their job, profession or rank, not by *who* they are. Being compassionate, however, is first of all acknowledging the other as a person, and that means going beyond dividing lines, differences and distinctions, even going against competitiveness.

Nouwen's (1982) book *Compassion* is based on the life of a doctor in Paraguay whose son was tortured to death. Through this the father had come to see compassion also as a political force by:

> defending the weak and indignantly accusing those who violate their humanity; joining with the oppressed in their struggle for justice; pleading for help with all possible means, from any person who has ears to hear and eyes to see.

Nurses are often in similar positions. By being advocates, taking independent decisions, by challenging management decisions, questioning treatments on the grounds of conscience (see Chapter 8) or values (see Chapter 3) nurses defend the weak and stand up with them against violations against humanity. But for this to be compassion, not just self-interest, we need to know from where this attribute comes, and what its aims are.

An interesting complementary point is made by Haughey (in Edwards, 1984) when he says that:

> the most compassionate thing you can do is 'know thyself'. Compassion is necessary where there are tensions. But to the extent that we do not know ourselves, we are continually making victims or inciting tensions that require others to be compassionate to those we have hurt, however unconsciously.

Compassions is more specific than caring. Compassion is 'questioning', 'resolving', 'joining', 'defending'. Caring calls forth caring; compassion 'manifests itself in critical situations' (Roach, 1985). Caring can be professional, but compassion has to be experienced. Caring can be learnt, but compassion comes out of the experience of having been hurt and having been shown compassion. We do not respond with compassion out of a sense of duty, but out of a sense of solidarity.

Competence

> Competence is a state of having the knowledge, judgment, skills, energy, experience and motivation required to respond adequately to the demands of one's professional responsibilities.

Competence distinguishes the practitioner from the student. It is that which every nurse longs for and works towards during basic and post-basic education and training.

Competence has also become a political issue in recent years. Clause 4 of the UKCC Code of Professional Conduct (see Chapter 5) states that a nurse who is asked to carry out delegated functions should acknowledge the limitations and refuse to carry out any such instructions if she or he is not competent. This is more than reasonable, yet these days the pressure is often intense – due mainly to shortness of staff – to go beyond the limit. In this sense, competence has become an issue of power and manipulation.

Roach warns that care will be diminished if competence becomes manipulation. She cites Fox (1979) who uses the symbol of the ladder: one who is climbing a ladder finds it more and more precarious, the higher he gets, to let go of the ladder and stretch out a hand to help others. The ladder becomes the focus; everything else becomes depersonalized.

Caring *does* demand competence, but competence with a human face. Care has to be appropriate, adequate, and practised with respect, considering the needs of those who are the recipients. In this way competence is very close to compassion; one tempers the other, one enhances the other by emphasizing that opposites need each other.

Confidence

Confidence is defined as the quality which fosters trusting relationships.

Most nurses would agree that at the basis of caring lies a trusting relationship. Without that the whole ethos of caring is lost.

Confidence is reciprocal; both parties in a relationship need to trust each other. But when one of the parties is in a professional position, then the other needs to be really sure that the professional can be trusted. This will depend largely on the degree of honesty (see Chapter 4) between them.

There is, today, a general erosion of confidence evident in most major institutions. People are wary of claims made by government, management of all kinds, advertising and the media. To counteract this, codes of practice seem to be proliferating among practitioners, and while they are welcome, they are nevertheless only as good as the people who use them.

If caring is to remain the unique feature of nursing, then confidence plays a large part. Genuine caring fosters confidence without coercion; it communicates truth without violence; and it creates relationships which are not paternalistic or based on fear or powerlessness, but are based on sharing and mutual respect.

Conscience

The word 'conscience' can be defined as a state of moral awareness; a compass directing one's behaviour according to the moral fitness of things.

Conscience is at the basis of ethical behaviour. Roach (1987) has a number of aphorism-like statements which help to explain this concept.

- 'Conscience is an intentional response, deliberate, meaningful and rational.'
- 'Conscience is the caring person attuned to the moral nature of things.'
- 'Conscience is the call of care and manifests itself as care.'
- 'Professional caring is reflected in a mature conscience.'

Conscience, as the faculty within, is learned from early childhood onwards and grows and develops. Parents and teachers instil a sense of right and wrong, and this eventually forms the value-basis on which judgements and decisions are made. Conscience is sometimes equated with 'feeling' – feeling bad about doing something. The feeling may very well be the indicator that something fundamental is at stake. The act of conscience then is the choice which directs the person in the better way.

The claim to conscience is so strong that most people would not go against it, or force anybody to go against their conscience. Conscience is a loyalty to oneself which should be respected in ourselves and in others as an innate right and as a duty in responding to something greater than ourselves. When conscience is allowed to be dulled or rationalized it can result in behaviour that may be less than admirable or excellent.

Because caring is essentially vulnerable, conscience is the element which directs a person into the right behaviour: the good, the creative and compassionate way of relating. It is perhaps the most spiritual of the 'Five Cs', and the one which demands the most constant attention.

Commitment

Commitment is:

> a complex affective response characterized by a convergence between one's desires and one's obligations, and by a deliberate choice to act in accordance with them.

If the Five Cs were along a line, commitment would come last. Commitment somehow confirms the other Cs. Similarly, the other attributes all have to be present for commitment to be viable.

The idea of commitment has been variously described also as devotion (Mayeroff, 1972), fidelity (May, 1975), and faithfulness (Häring, 1978). Campbell (1984a) says that 'consistent professional care is a form of love which entails a personal commitment by the person offering care'.

Commitment then, is that certain 'stickability' which gets a person involved with another person or in a task, without sentimentality or sense of burden. Commitment is a kind of response to a call which somehow is natural because caring is the human mode of being. Once the commitment is made – formally or informally, consciously at the time or only in retrospect – then it lasts for the duration of the relationship or the action, and it steers it positively.

This aspect of care is gaining in importance with the increased use of primary nursing. The ideal of that type of care rests on a commitment to the patient and the task by the primary nurse.

The care-giver

Caring is something practical, something done to some*one* by some*one*. Therefore we need to look at the persons who give and receive care. Books about nursing tend to concentrate on the patient and see the nurse only as the dispenser of care. Yet as the Five Cs show, that care-giver has to have a great deal of self-knowledge, self-understanding and self-assertiveness. Therefore to start with the nurse here seems logical.

A great deal has been written about self-awareness and how to achieve it (Bailey, 1985; Bond, 1986; Tschudin with Schober, 1990; Tschudin, 1991). The emphasis here is not so much on the *act* of self-awareness, as on what this eventually implies.

Caring involves for the care-giver first of all a 'feeling' with the other (Noddings, 1984). This is perhaps best captured in the word 'empathy', which basically means 'suffering-in'. Suffering is subjective; it is a 'feeling'. To understand suffering, a person has to be 'in'. It is not a question of *being* in the sufferer's shoes, nor even 'how would I feel in that position?'. It is a question of understanding the sufferer in her or his own position. It is not a question of projecting oneself into the other; it is a question of *receiving* the other into oneself. This may sound contrar to much that has been written about caring. On deeper reflection though, it can be seen that caring based on relationship can only be *received* caring. One cares for the other; one receives the other.

The philosopher Martin Buber (1937) has expressed the basic relationships which exist in terms of I and It, and I and Thou. I and It is the world of history, of objects and of the past. It is the world of things, and of experience, of perceiving, imagining, wanting, sensing and thinking.

The world of I and Thou is the world of relation: 'Whoever

says Thou does not have something; he *has* nothing. But he stands in relation.'

Buber describes how the word-set I–It appears as ego, that is, the I becomes conscious of itself, and of experience and use. In the word-set I–Thou, the I speaks as a person. *Egos* set themselves apart, but *persons* enter into relation with other persons. 'The purpose of relation is the relation itself – touching the (Thou). For as soon as we touch a (Thou), we are touched by a breath of eternal life.' As soon as there is a relation, there is something greater, something given.

This given is often expressed in nursing as job satisfaction. It is less the things given by the carer: the skills, the long hours, the tiredness, the unpleasant tasks, which matter. That is only what can be measured. What is received – what the patients give us: the appreciation of a relative, the smile of a sick child, knowing that you have 'been there' when it mattered – these are the reasons why nursing is so unique.

This sort of caring and being with another person is costly. Now the nursing process is a problem-solving approach to care. It is a logical, rational way of looking at care. When it was introduced it was hailed as the care-giver's solution to care. It has all the right questions and follows all the right steps.

But there is also another dimension. The carer is in relation with the care-receiver. That is what care is all about. The care-receiver has feelings about how and why she or he is washed, receives an injection, is told of a diagnosis, has treatments and plans discussed – or not. Anyone who has been at the receiving end of care will say that what matters most is how human the nurse or doctor – or any carer – is. Not how clever, how efficient, how good with the best equipment; no – but how able the carer is to receive the cared-for: that is what matters.

Caring *is* about process, and science, and detachment. And it is also about feeling – in-suffering – and about protecting and communicating. It is a kind of masculine approach which sees things in a linear way, and a feminine approach which sees things in a circular or spiral way. It is about giving and receiving. In order that the humanity of the persons concerned is not only maintained but enhanced, both masculine and feminine sides have to have their place in the scheme of things.

Caring has often been seen as giving, giving out, and sacrificing oneself. Caring was often also seen as dangerous, and nurses were warned not to 'get involved'. There are also plenty of people up and down the country who 'care' for a relative and who find this nothing but a chore. Sadly, that sort of care can neither give nor receive anything meaningful, but is a distortion of the whole concept of care which should be humanizing. But:

- How does a nurse care for a patient on dialysis who is also an alcoholic?
- How does a nurse care for a 'lifer', transferred to a hospital for intensive chemotherapy?
- How does a nurse care for an elderly person in her own home who is abusive and uncooperative, but will allow no one near her except the nurse?

Care can only be care when it is reciprocal. More than that, care has to be given to a *person* and received by a *person*. When the carer cannot give care in the way she or he would like to, she is diminished as a person. Equally, when the cared-for is not received by the carer as a person, the carer is diminished in her humanity. For care to be genuine, both people in the relationship have to be received. The main element of such receiving is listening.

Any care given may be competent, but if compassion, confidence or commitment are lacking, it is hollow care. This is where the carer's capacity for self-awareness and self-assessment is crucial. This is the work of conscience. Stepping back and examining what is happening, and perhaps taking stock of positions taken which might need to change: this is what receiving the other through listening is about.

Such self-searching is not easy. It can quickly become an inward-looking exercise which simply leads to more retrenched positions and one-sided views. The carer too needs care: she needs to be heard. Caring can only be given by a person who has also been heard. The person who cares for another who is overdemanding or unresponsive needs to be heard by someone else. Only thus is the circle of care closed. Or rather, it is a spiral which allows a person not just to go round and round, but up and down at the same side, seeing the problem from different levels.

Real caring demands a human person's fullest capacity to respond to the needs of another person, and in doing that there are sometimes situations which demand more than the usual, or catch us at unprepared moments, or at a time of personal struggle. These times and moments are challenges. To brush them aside – leaving your feelings at the door – is unrealistic and dehumanizing. We only become truly human, truly caring, *through* challenge, suffering, and suffering-in. But that has to be learnt, and sustained, and cared-for.

The care-receiver

In nursing one thinks of the one who receives care automatically as a patient. This basically implies someone static, ill, receptive. The term client gives a different idea: more like someone who shops for a particular article and pays for it. Neither of these terms are really satisfactory. And nurses are in close professional touch with the families and friends of those cared for, and with colleagues and indeed all those who make up the caring team. By using the term care-receiver the problem is not made easier, but it is intended to include all those with whom nurses are professionally in touch.

In our culture then, stress has been very heavily on giving: 'There is more happiness in giving than in receiving.' While we can teach how to give care, we usually don't teach how to receive; we just expect that people know how to do it when they are in a situation where they can't avoid it. This may actually be the wrong way round. Only when we know how to receive can we also give.

It can be argued that everyone knows how to receive because children receive their parents' care. Yet this cannot simply be taken for granted any more. And most adults suffer in life from some aspect or another of the care given or withheld, or given wrongly, by their parents. When they are then ill, or at some particular stage in life when they receive care, they may not know how to accept it. Equally, with the fragmentation of family life in society, some people – particularly elderly people – have become so independent that they reject any care which is well-meaning enough, but may be seen by them as an intrusion.

Yet other people may do just the opposite and squeeze every ounce of care out of the system and the people around them.

These are the extremes at both ends of the spectrum, but so that the norm can be seen more clearly, they have to be acknowledged too. In these instances, what is going on is not so much care-giving and receiving, but ego-tripping. The care-receiver is not able any more to say Thou to another, hence his or her I becomes isolated. Care in this instance, if solution-oriented, entirely misses the point, because it does not address the person.

The care which is person-oriented is very different. We have all been in situations when we felt that we were the only person in the whole world who mattered to someone. It was not just a giving and receiving of some*thing*, but a being together of two people. This implies that both were heard, and that hearing enhanced their humanity. It is out of such experiences that giving grows and becomes the sort of giving which selflessly enhances another.

This sort of giving should be the experience of the care-receiver. The cared-for is the only one who matters at this moment. He 'fills the firmament', as Noddings (1984) puts it. The care-giver is engrossed in the other. This presupposes an acceptance of the care-receiver which is non-judgemental.

When we are caring for a prisoner, or a cantankerous woman, we *are* judging them. We have to judge them in order to maintain our value-system, because they have forced us to question it. But in order to meet the person one needs to go beyond the appearance, beyond the misdeed, and particularly beyond one's fears and hang-ups; these are the things which block real care-giving and receiving more than the weightier matters of moral behaviour.

In Buber's term the other person is or becomes Thou. When we are really able to address a person as Thou – You – then we are with that person in a relationship which is not one-sided. We don't become overinvolved or absorbed in the other. When we truly say You to someone, we see that person as she or he is: autonomous, worthy of care and potentially healthy. It is so often in the paradox that we see the real situation; when I say You, truly, then I become I, truly. In giving the other his real self by saying You, I receive myself, because I have cared. But I cannot give of myself in order to receive; I give in order to give, and in doing that I receive.

The caring relationship

If, according to Buber, the one who says Thou to another, *has* nothing but stands in relation, then clearly that relationship is of utmost importance.

Using the images of masculine and feminine again, the masculine aspect of being human tends to isolation, to independence and to detachment. The feminine aspect of being human is more at home with 'receptivity, relatedness and responsiveness' (Noddings, 1984). This is that aspect which makes nursing unique. The caring done in nursing comes out of the sense of relating because something (someone) has been received. Noddings makes the further point that philosophers – who have been mostly men – start their theories with freedom ('Man' being an autonomous agent) and that that leads to an aloneness out of which one must act morally. The only thing felt in that situation is anguish; anguish at the responsibility which this aloneness and freedom brings. Women, on the other hand, experiencing relatedness, experience with that not anguish, but joy. This is a joy of being-with, of belonging and of receiving.

By making this point the masculine anguish is not denigrated, but rather highlights what has perhaps been obvious to many nurses: in caring we are fulfilled. This is equally true of men and women. In psychological terms a person is truly integrated when a man accepts the feminine aspects in himself and a woman accepts the masculine aspects in herself. In a caring relationship therefore both masculine and feminine play a part: the masculine capacity to separateness is as important as the feminine capacity for inclusion. If the feminine aspects are stressed more throughout this book, it is only because of the belief that in ethics in particular, the masculine – or perhaps just the male – has greatly dominated. To stress the feminine is therefore to redress a balance and to help legitimize some aspects of caring and nursing which have always been there but which may be in danger of being pushed aside by constant emphasis on masculine-oriented outlooks and theories.

The Five Cs of caring – compassion, competence, confidence, conscience and commitment – are only possible in a relationship. A person on a desert island would not be able to exercise any of these aspects, except perhaps towards animals, plants and ideas which, although they give us something, do not care for us by sharing any feelings with us. We come back then, to the point that caring rests on feelings. Where helping and caring are involved, these tend to be feelings of suffering – taking suffering in the widest sense. When caring is given from one human being to another human being, and relationship is created, then the main feeling which both are left with is joy. We are often too inhibited to call it joy, but feeling good, being cheerful, walking tall, job satisfaction, glowing with pride, as also the deep inner affirmation of having helped someone and knowing it – all these are aspects of joy.

A true relationship is not established on any rules. The nursing process sets certain standards, and so does an employing authority, the status of the carer, and the position of the care-receiver. When these limits and rules can be acknowledged *and* also set aside when necessary, then a relationship can happen.

The relationship between nurses and those they care for tends to start off very unequally: one is sick, one is healthy; one is ignorant, one is knowledgeable; one is receiving, one is giving. In many ways this has to be so in a world where expertise is becoming ever more necessary.

Sieghart (1985) points out that a 'professional' can only claim this title if he is willing to *share* his superior knowledge with his client. He puts his advantage at the disposal of the client. (A tradesman, in contrast, does what he is asked to do.) This has far-reaching ethical implications, in particular as regards informed consent (see Chapter 2). But this stance still implies that one is superior, another inferior.

Another view of this is taken by Campbell (1984a) who describes 'companionship'. The care-giver is a companion (the literal translation of the word means 'with-bread' – an evocative symbol) 'who shares freely, but does not impose, allowing others to make their journey'.

The people for whom nurses care in particular are all sick or injured – in body, mind or spirit – and those who surround them. Suffering is therefore the starting point. But the goal for all is a restoration to health or recovery (or a peaceful death). It is greater wholeness which we all strive for, nurses and patients, and in this we are one; in this we are not different. With these given things therefore, the relationship between care-givers and care-receivers is essentially directed already. But so that getting well is not just a process, like a necessary evil time one has to pass through, but a creative time, a caring relationship is necessary. The nurse who can help the patient to see this time of healing as a time of wider perspectives, of challenges and springboards to greater integrity and creativity is the nurse who is truly in touch with her or his own creativity. And creativity never happens alone: it always takes two – male and female (physically and/or metaphorically) to make something greater happen. When the care-giver is in touch with this and can call this creativity forth in the other, then there is relating and there is joy; in a sense then, the I is no more I, and the Thou is no more Thou, but *we* are now.

But is the care-receiver wanting to be in touch with such elements? Creativity is the most fundamental instinct of being human. This is not just procreation, but a creativity which is fruitful even when it is not fertile. It is a creativity which stems from a deep sense of needing to say Thou to something greater than ourselves, and therefore tends towards that Thou where alone it finds fulfilment. Health, or restoration to health, is part of this creativity, as is eventually a relinquishing of life so that the greater can come. Thus the care-receiver is in touch with all this, even if not always consciously.

This is put in philosophical terms because it needs to be said, somehow. The hallmark of a relationship though, is that it 'works'; two people have met and related. In that relating they cared and were cared-for; they gave care and received themselves. In whichever language it was expressed, what mattered is that I and Thou were both there, and that We have heard each other.

2

The caring relationship

Models of relationships

It is possible to see ethics in terms of ideals to be pursued. A caring relationship may therefore be an 'ideal' relationship. This does not diminish it; on the contrary, it is an ideal to strive for, and like a light leading the way.

In order to highlight the characteristics of an ethical relationship it is useful to look at various different ways in which relationships can be described.

Veatch (1972, in Aroskar, 1980b) has outlined four different types of relationships doctors have with patients: priestly, engineering, contractual and collegial models. These apply to nurses as well, particularly with the increase of primary nursing.

The priestly model

The priestly model is paternalistic. In this type of relationship the patient is passive, and the doctor or nurse 'plays God'. Any decision, particularly of an ethical nature, is the privilege or burden of the doctor, acting totally alone. The patient's values are not considered and not asked for. This model of a relationship is essentially unethical, as the patient's consent in matters which affect his life is not asked for. The exceptions are the 'incompetent' patients: the unconscious, the severely mentally handicapped or ill, and children below the age of consent.

The engineering model

In the engineering model the health care provider is seen to be the 'scientist'. The patient is given all the *facts*, so that he can then make his own choice. 'Health professionals become no more than plumbers cleaning out drains, as they service the wishes of patients.' This model of relationships is basically unsatisfactory, as neither the values nor the emotions of either patient or carer are taken into account, only the bare facts.

The contractual model

The contractual (contract, or covenant) model is very different. In this relationship the patient's values are explored and discussed. The nurse (or doctor) is of vital importance as a 'collaborator' on decisions to be taken.

This model is most closely allied to the concept of caring. It is also essentially the model advocated by the nursing process. It shows a respect for the person, and is built on a relationship of sharing, enhancing each other and respecting each other's needs and values.

The collegial model

The collegial model is highly idealistic. Both patient and nurse share mutual goals and act as 'pals'. Decisions are reached by consensus. However, even Veatch agrees that this model is rather impractical.

A different approach to relationships is taken by May (1975). He distinguishes between relationships characterized by code, covenant, contract or philanthropy.

Code

A code shapes human behaviour and practitioners of any profession stand or fall by them. They remain practitioners largely by self-discipline in keeping the code. A professional relationship which is based mainly on the idea of keeping a code is on the whole clearcut. Involvement with patients or clients is not encouraged as the code regulates professional life only, and compassion – 'suffering with' – infringes on the professional's private commitments. This can be seen clearly in the way duty hours are regulated, home telephone numbers are not given to clients and until recently the title 'nurse' protected a practitioner's personal name.

Covenant

A covenant always has a reference to a 'specific historical exchange between partners leading to a promissory event'. 'Covenant ethics is responsive in character.' A covenant has a gift as its basis which both sides experience. There is a covenant promise involved based on this gift. The subsequent life of both parties is shaped by this promise of gift. Translated into nursing terms, this means that the nurse gives of her or his skill and professional experience to help the patient in whichever way this is appropriate. But this is not a detached helping. The nurse gives of herself and himself. Thus a relationship is formed. The covenant means that the relationship is between two *people*, not just between an expert and an inexpert. The future for both parties is shaped by this event (most patients remember their nurses!) because they communicate and respond to each other, creating and so co-creating each other's lives.

Contract

A contract is recognized by its need for informed consent. The notion of a contract includes an exchange of information on the basis of which an agreement is reached. This relates to the 'engineering model' above.

As informed consent is the central concern of this model, it may be useful to look at it in some more detail here.

Informed consent

The notion of informed consent stems from the 1947 Nuremberg Trials of twenty-three Nazi doctors accused of crimes involving human subjects. The Nuremberg Code (1947) lays down ten standards to which doctors must conform when carrying out experiments on human subjects. Voluntary consent of the subject is the first of these standards. (The Nuremberg Code is now largely replaced by the Declaration of Helsinki (1964); see Chapter 5.)

The idea of consent is based on the principle of respect for the person, and thus on the concept of human rights (or 'natural law') of life and liberty.

In recent years it has become increasingly clear that consent is more than the required signature on a piece of paper prior to going to surgery. In her book *Whose Body Is It?* Carolyn Faulder (1985) describes informed consent as 'the right to know' and as 'the right to say no'.

The right to know 'must come from a full explanation of the nature, purpose, duration, methods, means, inconveniences, hazards and possible effects' (Anon. 1988) of all treatments, invasive or otherwise, and of all experiments. Why this is not always done is easy to see: those offering treatments are experts who cannot expect that those who come to them for help are in a position to understand as much as they, nor can they be given *all* the information to make a truly educated, or responsible, decision. That is not what is in doubt. What is questioned far more often is that some information is not given, or is deliberately given in such a way that the client cannot understand, as when using medical terms or abbreviations.

Equally often the complaint is that patients who are entered in research trials are not told of these.

Faulder's 'right to say no' is affected here. When a patient can say no to such experiments or being part of a trial, then this can adversely affect the trial.

Nurses are more and more involved in the setting up and running of experiments and trials of all kinds. They often assist doctors by keeping records of blood pressure, taking blood, or monitoring mental states of patients. When patients know what is happening all is well, but if they find that they are being treated differently from other patients and begin to be suspicious, the difficulties arise.

Essentially, all nursing actions are invasions of a person's privacy. Most of these actions are considered necessary and consent is given implicitly by going into hospital, or being treated at home. This should, however, never be taken for granted. Giving full explanations of what is being done and why, how, where and when, is essential for the patient or client to remain a free agent and exercise the right to say no.

Nurses are often in a quandary of not knowing what their obligations are with regard to information-giving to patients. Clearly, a surgeon needs to explain an operation and a physician other types of treatments. But then the patient thinks over what this all means and asks the nurse to elaborate, or explain again.

- Can the nurse add information the patient does not seem to have?
- Can the nurse outline any options, or point to alternative treatments which the doctor has not given?
- What burdens does this put on the patient?
- What ethical problems does this create for the nurse vis-à-vis the doctor?

These are weighty points which will be elaborated on in the next chapter.

The legal aspect of consent is based on 'competence'. Children under the age of sixteen are not able to give consent but their parents or guardians have to give it on their behalf. Mentally handicapped or ill people pose a much greater problem, as do people who are temporarily or permanently rendered unconscious or otherwise unable to communicate. These are the cases which then often come to law, as for instance *In Re B* (*IME Bulletin*, 1987a). B was a mentally retarded girl of seventeen in the care of Sunderland Borough Council. The council had applied for an order to make her a ward and for leave to have her sterilized. This was supported by her mother. The case went back and forth in the law. Was her welfare and best interest served by preventing pregnancy which would be an 'unacceptable risk'? (This is a deontological view. The teleological view would take into consideration also the long-term consequences this decision might have for similar cases: see Chapter 4.)

Four basic elements always have to be considered in consent:

- Who may give consent.
- The competency of the individual.
- Who should provide the information.
- The content of the information.

It is interesting that the root of the word consent means 'to feel together'. Consent is not just a legal need, but a caring act which involves relating to one another.

After this lengthy incursion into informed consent, the other aspects of May's models are resumed.

Philanthropy

May is ruthless about this approach: it is condescending, gratuitous (rather than responsive or reciprocal) and conceited. This model is imitating God. Philanthropy here equates with the priestly model above.

In Veatch's model the contractual ideal is seen as the really worthwhile and workable approach. May goes a step further by declaring that neither code nor contract are basic to human (that is, creative and healing) relationships, but covenants are: in them something is freely given and freely *responded* to.

In all relationships there are possibilities for abuse and difficulties. Benjamin and Curtis (1986) see these among nurses mainly to be based around the issues of paternalism, deception and confidentiality. (Confidentiality will be dealt with in Chapter 8.)

Paternalism

Paternalism – or 'parentalism' as Benjamin and Curtis prefer to call it – is frowned upon nowadays, yet in many ways it still thrives. The automatic use of first names, and calling people 'Pop' and 'Sweetie' may sound harmless enough, but it does point to an air of superiority. It may even indicate a kind of disrespect as it usually comes from young nurses to older patients.

Patients may often be glad, at least for a while, not to have to make decisions; they may not be able to think straight because they are too shocked; they don't know much about anatomy, physiology or chemistry; they are rightly afraid of unknown therapies and treatments, including operations, and unless they have experience, they cannot judge outcomes and prognoses. But that doesn't mean that they do not think or have no feelings. Doctors have often told patients 'We (using the plural) will do this . . . ', and nurses have followed the custom, without so much as a 'by your leave'. This causes understandable resentment on behalf of the patients. Care based on a relationship is helping to eliminate this difficulty. But like all forms of discrimination, it is subtle, inbred and difficult to challenge.

An example of blatant paternalism is related by Duncan, Dunstan and Welbourne (1981) where in 1952 the law had in fact defended a lie 'for the patient's good'.

> A surgeon told a patient about to be operated on for goitre that the operation carried no risk to her voice. He knew in fact that there was some risk but said that there was none in order not to cause the patient distress. At operation damage was caused and the patient sued for negligence. At trial the judge, in summing up, declared that what the surgeon had said had been for the patient's good and was in the circumstances justifiable. The surgeon was acquitted.

This condescending and gratuitous attitude is unlikely to be defended today, but it is far from gone completely.

Deception

Deception is no less difficult a subject. Deception, say Benjamin and Curtis (1986) 'is a form of manipulation, and manipulation, like coercion and rational persuasion, is a way of inducing others to do what one wants them to do'.

One reason for so much routine in nursing work is to make life easier for nurses by making patients compliant. Although it may often not be admitted, nurses sometimes 'punish' patients who are not readily compliant, by withholding information or services from them.

> David was a 27-year-old man with AIDS. He was the leader of a band, and his lifestyle was somewhat unusual in that he slept until late in the day and was awake most of the night. He was not willing, on his frequent short hospitalizations, to change this style. Thus he asked for his breakfast at about 3 p.m. When, at 8 p.m., he had not had his 'lunch' for two days running, he asked his nurse for it. He said he had 'forgotten' to bring it to him. The staff had in fact decided not to give it to him as one way of teaching him to 'toe the

line'.

- Are such tactics either realistic or ethical?
- What should be done if 'the required behaviour does not occur: a little more starvation?'. (Flanagan, 1986)

Conflicting claims

This often ties in with deception. When a nurse does not know who has the greatest claim on her time, skill, or attention, she or he may have to resort to manipulative or underhand practices. The patient often has the greatest claim, but various members of the family – particularly in the case of child-patients – or doctors make equally strong claims on nurses' professional and emotional capacities.

> Harry was eleven when he was admitted with a painful and swollen left leg, diagnosed as sarcoma. Harry lived with his younger sister and recently divorced mother. On the ward he was quiet but watched every game of football and rugby on the television. His mother had been adamant that Harry should not be told anything of his prognosis and the consultant had agreed to this. Harry had suffered quite enough already, she said. Clare, a student nurse, became very friendly with Harry and he asked her more and more questions about his leg, which she found increasingly difficult to answer because of the proviso not to tell him anything. She asked that this 'don't tell policy' should be reversed, but the consultant felt he couldn't let Harry's mother down. Clare decided she could not maintain her integrity under these circumstances and asked to be transferred to another ward. Harry became quiet and withdrawn again and died three weeks later.

It need not only be children who have the truth kept from them. The priestly or philanthropic models of relationship are often used as a way out of a difficult situation of communication. It tends to be the nurses who are then in the tight corner. Their loyalty is to the patient, because they are *for* him or her, but they are also *for* the family, a unit which may have functioned for years in a particular way that they have no right to destroy.

In a case conference discussed by Higgs (1985) of a situation similar to that of Harry, most of the commentators suggested that the adults (parents and doctors) should be given an opportunity to voice their fears, angers and worries. The point was made strongly that: 'When we think we can tell them what's wrong, then we're missing the point. We have to find out what they are worried about... One has to understand *that* by listening to (them) and not spend hours talking *at* (them).' An ethic of caring essentially listens.

The difficulties between nurses and patients are usually communication problems. They arise because of prior personal problems of insecurity and inexperience leading to aggressive or manipulative behaviour. But such difficulties then become violations of ethical principles, particularly of truth-telling, justice and freedom (see Chapter 4). What happens to one person will eventually happen to many.

- Is it right that personal problems encroach on professional relationships?
- What does creativity in caring relationships mean in practice?
- What can a nurse do when she or he sees deception, and paternalism going on around her or him?

The 'new nursing'

The term 'new nursing' was coined by Salvage (1990) to describe an internal reform movement which she believes dates back to the early 1970s and is basically an ideology of partnership.

The background to this movement can be sketched in a few broad outlines.

Without doubt, the introduction of the nursing process had started a revolution in nursing. The task-oriented approach gave way to the patient-oriented approach. This was further highlighted when nursing models came onto the scene. These new ways of working demanded of nurses to ask some fundamental questions about care and the relationships between themselves and patients, and between themselves and doctors. It was not so much a question any more of what is a nurse, or what do nurses do, but: what is nursing? The answers have to do with 'receptivity, relatedness and responsiveness' (Noddings, 1984) pointing to values, to meaning and to community. Practically, this is characterized by assertiveness among nurses and a move away from the disease-oriented medical model to a holistic model of care.

Movements towards equality between the sexes in pay, status, education and job opportunities have fostered an assertiveness which is unknown for many people. Nurses have often been portrayed as angels, handmaids, sex symbols or domineering matrons; and they have colluded with these images. As assertiveness grows in strength these stereotypes lose their hold. Nurses don't have to project an image any longer in order to be accepted or taken seriously. But assertiveness does not come easily after a long time of submissive 'second fiddler' status.

With some of these influences in the background, Salvage believes that two opposing ideologies advocate partnership: those who draw on the ideals of humanistic psychology and the one-to-one relationship; and those who defend the market forces and competitive strategies. Basically, both sides are about power relations. Where nurses see themselves as partners, however, the need for power and defence of power is diminished drastically.

The new nursing is practised as such in very few places. Where it is practised, and nurses are in charge rather than doctors, the effects are drastic. The traditional hierarchy is not needed; a primary nurse enters a partnership with the patient and according to one study: 'patients...received better and more consistent care...; became more independent; were more satisfied with their nursing; were generally as satisfied with life; had a shorter average stay in acute care; and incurred lower average costs! A surprise finding was the statistically significant reduction in the death rate of...patients while in hospital, compared with (a) control group.'

Salvage makes the point that many patients judge the quality of nursing by its 'emotional style'. She is not alone in this: the many care studies in the nursing press week by week put increasing emphasis on this aspect of care. Patients neither expect nor want a quasi-psychotherapeutic relationship with the nurse, but look for 'warmth, kindness and sensitivity'. The partnership is thus based on the human needs presented – relief from pain and discomfort – but the way in which this is done is significant. 'Any nurse can stick a needle or an enema into anything human, and for that matter into beings which are not human. But not all nurses can supply optimum care (...) to all patients' (Jourad, 1971).

The idea of partnership with the patient or client stems from the sense of 'being in this together' – a sense of a common destiny. The individual (I) who becomes or is more assertive – does not care for any self-gain. The individual cares for another (Thou). Real care is always other-directed. Real care is also more than just helping to heal a broken limb by keeping the traction functioning. Real care is helping the *person* to adjust to the broken limb and then adjust his or her life to that new situation, and finally integrate the whole event into the wider context of health and illness. Some patients do this with ease and seemingly without thinking about it; others need help, particularly if the illness is a serious one, or threatens the person's livelihood. This is where the caring role of nurses is such a significant one. Their competence and experience, their compassion and commitment is vital – though often not demonstrative – in helping clients and patients to make sense of their illness and limitations. A nurse is more than just the critical link with the outside world in a hospital, but often also the link for a patient between his or her external situation and internal experience.

Sadly, Salvage (1990) concludes that not many nurses either do, or are inclined to, care in a partnership way. The patient-centred care is eroded by 'staff shortages, lack of time, the bureaucratic management system employed by most ward sisters, a mixture of organizational constraints and the emotional safety or routine work'.

Yet the increasing trend to have primary nursing, more care in the community, a slowly increasing understanding of patient-centred care and the introduction of Project 2000 all contribute to more partnership. The model of disease-orientation is giving way to a model of person-orientation, where 'life' is seen as a whole. Disease, disability, old age and death are perceived less as 'bad' and enemies to be fought against, but are considered again as part of life and living. But this is not without its problems. Increasing technology is not increasing bliss. The more we know, the more we have to use this knowledge responsibly. Technology and knowledge can lead to increasing independence – but also isolation. The new nursing with its emphasis on partnership is ideally placed consciously to balance this by the way it treats its 'partners' in 'receiving' them, relating to them and responding to them with care. In that way it is ideally a covenant relationship based on the gift of self.

3

Values and value-statements

Values

Values are the personal aspects and foundations of social and ethical living. Values are deep and very important, like the value a person places on the house to live in, or having certain friends. But they can also be more superficial, like the clothes one wears, or a certain food one eats. Yet that in itself is making a value-statement: for some people these very things could be the other way round. What is important to one may be valueless to another.

Values are here to help us choose between alternatives, make decisions, and resolve conflict.

Values can be divided into three levels of expressions: beliefs, attitudes and values themselves.

Beliefs

A belief is probably the most basic value and the one that changes least. A belief is a type of attitude which is based more on faith than fact. Anne Frank (1958) wrote in her diary that 'people are really good at heart' three weeks before being captured by the Nazis and deported to a concentration camp where she died.

A belief goes beyond the obvious, but it starts from the basis of some fact at least. One needs to have met some people who are good at heart in order to believe that all – or most of them – are good at heart.

Perhaps one of the main beliefs in nursing is that patients will get better with good care. Another belief may be that this, rather than other work, is ultimately satisfactory.

Attitudes

An attitude is a disposition, or a settled behaviour. Attitudes are rather constant feelings, usually made up of different beliefs.

Some of the attitudes particular to nursing are expressed in the way care is given. Henderson (1966) describes the 'unique function of a nurse' in her now famous statement. The second part of that is: 'The nurse is temporarily the consciousness of the unconscious, the love of life of the suicidal, the leg of the amputee, the eyes of the newly blind, a means of locomotion for the newborn, knowledge and confidence for the young mother, a voice for those too weak to speak, and so on.'

These are 'functions' which a nurse performs, but without the attitudes based on the beliefs that they are valuable, no nurse could simply perform these functions. Moreover, Henderson believes that these are unique to nursing and that no other health workers would claim them or take them from nurses. Thus the attitudes with which they are performed are also unique to nursing.

Values

Values are less fixed, and more dynamic, than beliefs and attitudes because there is usually an element of motivation involved.

Raths, Harmin and Simon (1966) believe that people who are (or appear to be) flighty, apathetic, moody, rebellious, conforming and submissive, or phoney, may be people who have not come to grips with their own values.

Frankl (1962) argued that the most important goal in life for each person is the search for meaning. A person finds meaning through values. Frankl speaks of three types of values: creative, experiential and attitudinal.

Creative values

Creative values are those which are discovered through what we do, particularly through helping others. Any job can in this sense be seen as helping someone to discover some values. Being a shop assistant is creative: it is being of value to someone and it creates income. Cooking is creative: it is necessary for keeping alive, and it also keeps the family together when eating, or it is in preparation for a party or celebration of some event. It is clear that nursing as a job will give more satisfaction than working on a conveyor belt. Helping people in any kind of way will always highlight some values; being of use to others strengthens the sense of self-worth, increases relationships and widens the emotional and intellectual horizon. Simply making a patient comfortable in bed gives a sense of achievement, but having relieved another person's distress means that a human need has been responded to, and that is what living is most deeply about.

Experiential values

Experiential values are those which are discovered through appreciation of people, events and natural or artistic beauty.

Frankl points out that values cannot be *created* – they are discovered. We do not set out to make ourselves happy. We do something like going to a concert and the appreciation of the music makes us happy. A wonderful sunset or the sight of Niagara Falls can give one a sense of awe and wonder and put one in touch with nature or with the infinite. These then become values and one may set out to experience them again. Before they were experienced for the first time, they may have been known *about* but not known to oneself, nor would one know if one would or should choose them for oneself.

The same is true of values about people. An honest person is known when meeting one, and that heightens the sense of the importance of honesty. People like Martin Luther King, Mother Theresa of Calcutta, or Margaret Thatcher stand for certain ideals. One can accept these ideals or leave them, but the experience one has of the value of their ideals is important. But it is not only the great and the good who inspire. A dying child, a sick father and any 'ordinary' patient can lead nurses to discover values by being around them, i.e. by 'experiencing' these people for what they are and who they are.

Attitudinal values

Attitudinal values are those which are discovered through the way in which one reacts to unfortunate circumstances over which there is no control, such as one's own and other people's suffering.

Frankl's main theory is that people need to have a meaning in life, and that their task is to search for this meaning. Thus illnesses, accidents and suffering of all kinds are triggers in that search, and sometimes the answer itself.

Anyone who has an accident or a serious illness will ask at some stage: Why? Why me? Why now. Why in this way? These questions, and the answers finally given to them, shape a person's life. When a person has discovered the meaning in life, then he or she lives purposefully. The way in which a person who is ill is cared for will inevitably contribute to the discovery of meaning in life.

Values only take on significance when they are tested against someone or something. We may say that we value life, but it is probably only after brushing with death through an illness or an accident that we truly appreciate our own life.

Nursing values only become relevant when they are questioned. When the question, 'What does this situation mean?' is asked a person becomes aware that there may be a right and a wrong. In the days when nurses were bidden not to ask questions, there were few values. Now the reverse is true: nurses need to ask questions and are asked them, therefore they need to be aware also of their values.

This may feel and sound disconcerting. Just as certain values seem to be established, they are challenged and discarded. Cupitt (1990) thinks that this points to the fact 'that everything is invented and all our highest and most precious beliefs and values are mere cultural fictions'. If this is so, it also points to 'the necessity of devising authoritative new beliefs and values that will more strictly control our economic activities than ever the sincerely-held dogmatic religion of the past succeeded in doing'.

This then points to the danger that some authority simply replaces one set of values with another and the people affected gain little except perhaps a different vocabulary. The challenge then is to question the authority: how paternalistic, covenantal or contractual is it? Can it be trusted and should it be trusted? How paternalistic would a rival authority be? These may be rhetorical questions, but they do crop up a great deal in all areas of life.

One hundred value-statements

Table 3.1 is a list of 100 general value-statements. They are meant simply to make readers more aware of what values are, and what they may mean. It may be possible to read this list and mark which statements have greatest (G), medium (M) or lowest (L) value for any reader.

Table 3.1   Value-statements. Reprinted from Simmons (1982), with permission of the author

1   The opportunity to improve my standard of living
2   Owning my own house
3   Having modern conveniences like a deep freeze or automatic washing machine
4   Having good health
5   Living to a happy old age
6   Having an adequate social security system
7   Being successful in my work
8   Having happy, healthy children
9   Being part of a happy family
10   Preserving social justice
11   Fighting for what I believe in
12   Being open and sincere
13   The state of ecstasy
14   The state of tranquility
15   Having a close pair relationship
16   Being private
17   Being physically fit
18   The pleasure of being with others
19   Being the one who always brings about change
20   Fighting to preserve the natural world
21   Resisting the pressures to be or do something which is against my will
22   Developing new ways of living in the modern world
23   Maintaining the tried and true ways of living which have proved right
24   Approaching the solution of social problems with unrestrained zeal
25   Resolving social disputes through calm diplomacy
26   Moderation in all moods
27   A closeness with my own inner self

Table 3.1 *continued*

28 Being open and receptive to others
29 Enjoying sensual experiences with relish and abandonment
30 Faith in God
31 Continually and actively striving towards some end
32 Experiencing an empathy for all ways of life
33 Floating along in a casual and carefree state of existence
34 Always being in control of my experiences
35 Overcoming or conquering some obstacle
36 Seeking adventure and excitement
37 The joy of humility and cooperativeness which aids others to become more themselves
38 Appreciating the beauty of a work of art
39 Creating an object of beauty
40 Making a contribution to basic knowledge
41 Thinking ideas and enjoying thoughts
42 The hope of being wealthy
43 Participating in the business life of the community
44 Being a part of political activities
45 Being in charge of the lives of others
46 Spending my time organizing and directing
47 Entertaining others
48 Spending my time at parties
49 Being recognized for my accomplishments
50 The opportunity to become a celebrity
51 Being of service to others
52 Being as charitable as possible
53 Living a comfortable life
54 Leading a meaningful life
55 Working for a world of peace
56 Having equality among all people
57 Leading a life of freedom
58 Being a mature person
59 Living in a secure nation
60 Respecting others
61 Being respected by others
62 Achieving salvation
63 Achieving wisdom
64 Experiencing true friendship
65 Loving my parents
66 Becoming aware through demonstrating/protesting
67 Developing and maintaining a career for myself

Table 3.1 *continued*

68	Establishing and maintaining a marriage and family
69	Defending the oppressed
70	Maintaining a democratic society
71	Caring for my parents
72	Avoiding an adherence to any ideology
73	Being generous
74	Being well-dressed
75	Controlling my own impulses so they don't get out of hand
76	Following rules which I accept
77	Avoiding idleness
78	Avoiding anarchy through a strong central government
79	Achieving a sense of community and belonging together with all people
80	Being a decent, normal person
81	Developing myself into a more satisfying person
82	Feeling like a worthwhile person
83	Leading a disciplined life
84	Being thrifty
85	Accepting circumstances for what they are
86	Becoming aware of the potential for change around me
87	Developing or discovering means to change the world in which we live
88	Truth
89	Goodness
90	Order
91	Being unique
92	Simplicity
93	Justice
94	Playfulness
95	A sense of everything being connected
96	Loyalty
97	Accepting the inevitable
98	Being victorious
99	Being myself
100	Purity

This list is by no means complete. When thinking about values, such a list simply gives an idea of what is actually involved.

Simon and Clark (1975, in Steele and Harmon, 1983) suggest that people arrive at their own values through choosing, prizing and then acting on them. For a value to be really owned a person needs to have the freedom to acquire it. There must also be the freedom to choose from alternatives, all of which must be able to be considered thoughtfully. A person needs to know why he or she has chosen this particular value, then it needs to be prized and cherished, and one must be willing to make it known to others. Lastly, a person then needs to behave in such a way as to show that a choice has been made; in other words, the value must be integrated into action.

This book suggests that caring is such a value. In choosing to become a nurse, a person chooses to care. Each person expresses this differently, but one can care either because one has to, or because one wants to. How each person expresses care will not only be a personal moral or ethical choice, but it will be expressed in relationship with others, particularly in the way other people's values are respected.

Values are dynamic. Young people see most things in terms of right and wrong, black and white. Experiences of life, mixing with people and discerning meaning, shape and change one's values. The process of choosing, prizing and acting on is therefore a constantly repeating one. For some people more and more things have value; others feel that as they get older fewer and fewer values emerge.

Values that are repeatedly threatened in ethics are those related to the value of life itself (Steele and Harmon, 1983). In the setting of nursing, the values of care, of health and of health care also have a particular place.

Values of caring

In saying that caring is the human mode of being, Roach (1987) also says that caring is a response to someone or something who or which matters. The response is 'to value as the important-in-itself'. And 'value does not seek further proof other than that it is: it is self-evident'. There is no question that a person or pet, or sunset exists; she, he or it simply *is*, and in order to be truly human, the response is to her, him or it from that human point of view. This shows clearly the elements of caring outlined in Chapter 2:

- *Receptivity* – the other is received as she, he or it is.

- *Relatedness* – receiving someone or something means to be in relation to her, him or it.
- *Responsivity* – receiving alone is not enough; receiving comes alive through responding. The person who responds calls forth a response in the other, and thus a relationship is created.

With these values of relating need to be put Roach's (1987) Five Cs as values of caring (see Chapter 1):

- Compassion
- Competence
- Confidence
- Conscience
- Commitment

The following story may help to put these abstract terms into the perspective of caring practice.

> I remember in my nursing days having to care for a middle-aged man suffering from multiple sclerosis. F was rather overweight and much misunderstood. He had been moved from a medical to a geriatric ward because 'he was taking up too much of the nurses' time in an acute medical ward'. 'He's always moaning and complaining', I was told. I was on night duty on the senior citizens' ward when I first met F. In helping him to retire at night, I was constantly helping him to change his position. Every few minutes of the first half hour, he would ask for his position to be changed, 'move my leg, move my arm, move my buttock,' he would say. It was always move this, move that, and he could be quite trying. However, I soon learned that if I took time to listen and hear F and move him as and when he requested, it could mean spending 20–30 minutes with him.
>
> But then finally, he would say, 'I'm fine now, thank you.' He would soon be asleep and would invariably sleep through the whole night. It was only when I could feel his pain, his helplessness, through hearing and paying full attention to his requests that F was able to sleep securely. This, I am sure, was because attention was being paid to him as a person rather than as a patient. It enabled him to feel that

he was still valuable enough for someone to listen to him and to affirm him as a person who happened to be labelled a patient.

F taught me a great deal about having the patience not only to listen but, more importantly, how to hear. He also taught me how difficult it is to take time to listen to the pain of another who is constantly complaining that no one understands and that no one cares that he is full of pain. He needed me and my time to listen to the meaning of his pain. Naturally this is difficult when you have 20–30 other persons in the ward demanding the presence of your ears. (Kirkpatrick, unpublished)

Together with this story and the values outlined above need to be put also some more general points. Rogers (1961) has listed some principles of helping which, when applied to caring, become values.

Being

Before we can *do* we need to *be*: be ourselves, one human person with another human person. This entails that we *are* trustworthy, honest, dependable.

Clarity

A willingness to *be* expresses itself in a clarity towards the other. We say what we think of this relationship. If we feel uneasy we say so, otherwise the relationship may be harmed by playing games with each other.

Respect

We do not always like someone at first sight. But in caring we respect a person, and this may lead to a mutual liking.

Separateness

Even though we are caring, and deeply caring, we are not engulfed by the other, downcast by his depression, or frightened by his fear. We need to remain a separate person.

Freedom

The other person needs to be free to express himself or herself and be what he or she is even though we may not like some types of freedom.

Empathy

This is the ability to perceive the feelings of the other person, and the ability to communicate this to him or her (Kalisch, 1971). When we can understand what goes on within ourselves then we may be able to understand the world of the other better.

Communication

Both our verbal and non-verbal communication should convey that we are 'for' this person. What we convey should correspond to what is relevant and encouraging.

Evaluation

Evaluation of a situation helps, but all too often we use and take evaluation personally. In caring we need to be clear and specific, as does the other person. When we help a person to evaluate where she is in relation to where she has come from and where she wants to go, then we care for and about her.

Becoming

All caring is so that the other can grow and become. 'I can recognize in him the person he has been created to become. I confirm him in myself, and then in him, in relation to this potentiality that can now be developed, can evolve' (Buber, 1957, in Rogers, 1961).

As caring is a human act, human feelings and behaviour characterize it. When these are positive and helpful, caring takes place. But all is not always as rosy as that. Breakdown of relationships happens; feelings of anger, resentment, hate and destruction are often more powerful than their good opposites. The Five Cs would in the past have been called virtues. 'Virtue' is not a word which rolls easily off the tongue these days. Calling the Five Cs values may give them a less emotive image. Yet it is not the practice of virtue*s* which matter, but of virtu*e*, i.e. integrity (MacIntyre, 1985). Anger, fear, resentment and so on are legitimate and often helpful feelings. It is when they are used with integrity that the other feelings of love, joy and peace can also stand as outcomes of caring.

Values of health

The values of health are far from simple. The World Health Organization (WHO, 1947) definition of health is 'a state of complete mental, physical and social well-being and not merely the absence of disease or infirmity'. While such documents have to aim high, it can be asked, who is *completely* mentally, physically and socially healthy? A condition can be a minor irritation for one person but a serious illness for another. This can be seen even in cultural quirks: the British tend to be concerned about 'being regular', the French about their 'crise de foie', and the Germans about their 'Herzkrise' (Swaffield, 1990a).

The different emphasis which different groups of people put on health may be illustrated by the following story.

> Mr W had had a laryngectomy for carcinoma of the larynx when he was fifty-eight. This left him with a permanent tracheostomy. Mr W had been a heavy smoker all his life, and after the operation continued with the practice, smoking through the tracheostomy. Doctors and nurses tried every means to dissuade him from smoking, and the family did the same, occasionally threatening him, but all to no avail. When two years later there was fresh evidence of carcinoma in the region, the oncologist gave Mr W an ultimatum: either he stop smoking, or he would not give him any treatment.

Clearly, the values of doctors and patients often differ.

In his 'Reith Lectures' Sacks (1990) made the point that without objective standards we have no coherent language of ethics. We have largely lost a sense of obligations which constrain our choices, and duties which put limits on our desires. We are much more aware of 'autonomy, equality and rights – the values that allow each of us to be whatever we choose'. 'Thus,' he argues, 'we choose our own acts freely; but we believe that the consequences should be dealt with by the state. Thus we have the almost impossible situation where governments are there to treat AIDS, child abuse, homelessness and addiction but cannot, or should not, disseminate a morality that might reduce them in the first place.' There are no objective standards applicable to all, and therefore the language of one group of people offends that of another.

Care and cure are not value-free. To think otherwise is 'malignant nonsense' according to Illich (1976). In the years since Illich wrote, this has become even more evident.

Most values concerning health are based on perceived need:

- What is the person's bodily or mental need? The patient thinks, for example, she needs vitamins; the doctor disagrees.
- What is the goal of the need? What state of health could be reached with care or treatment? The patient may look for complete restoration; the doctor thinks differently – or vice versa.
- A patient may not agree that certain secondary effects of treatments are acceptable; the doctor may think that a requested treatment is not worthwhile.

The perceived needs for, and in, health depend largely on the theories or concepts about health which a person holds. Liss and Nordenfelt (1990) point out that in an analytical framework of health statistical normality is the key concept, whereas a holistic theory views a whole person's function and activity. The values which arise from either of these approaches will colour the stance taken. The above statements look different depending on which theory either party holds. The fact is that 'both the goal of need and the suitable treatment to reach the goal are things we choose' (Liss and Nordenfelt, 1990).

The choices of either party in this scenario are based on values which have been accumulated over the years with experience. A person who had one 'bad' operation may put up with considerable discomfort before even contemplating having another operation. A doctor who has seen many patients with similar conditions will think it practically impossible for someone not to undergo a certain treatment despite 'a few' side-effects.

A very broad generalization can perhaps be made here about these views. A more masculine approach is to see life and problems in terms of progression from A to B; in statistics, symptoms and prognoses. A more feminine view would be to see health in terms of all-inclusive functioning and well-being. Women may be more likely to live with 'imperfection' in terms of health, and talk not of cure but of healing. This could point to the often opposing stance taken by nurses and doctors with regard to health and the patients they care for. Yet without the analytical approach medicine would not be where it is today. Without the more holistic approach medicine cannot survive. It may be that at this moment in time nurses need to affirm positively the more specifically feminine view of health in order to redress the balance.

Values of health care

It is a truism that every aspect of health care is constantly changing. What applies today may not apply tomorrow. Some things written in this book may be outdated by the time it is read.

The values which apply to caring all begin with 'C'; those which apply to health care all seem to begin with 'E':

- Economy
- Efficiency
- Effectiveness

At least, these are the guidelines which the Audit Commission is applying to Health Authorities, self-governing trusts and Family Practitioner Committees to find out if they give value for money (Hodges, 1990).

Most of western society is committed to a capitalist system which is based on the idea of the market. Goods should be freely available and the customer has the choice of what to buy. This is also increasingly the norm for health care. The 'customer' should be free to choose which treatment to have where and when. This presupposes that the customer is well informed about choices available, is in a position mentally and emotionally to make these choices, has the cash resources to pay for them, and that the treatments chosen are available where and when they are wanted or needed. There are two big difficulties with this in

Britain: the NHS does not function as a market at present; and not all people, in fact only very few, have the financial resources to buy health care as on a market. An ever-widening gap of inequality is therefore appearing.

There are stories without number of people who were refused treatment or given inappropriate treatments for questionable reasons:

- A 'gentleman of the road' being refused kidney dialysis (Gaze, 1985).
- A 15-year-old boy who, at the end of his tether and strength with chemotherapy for a rare form of leukaemia had pulled out his Hickman line, had it inserted again against his will.
- A 45-year-old mother of five young children being told that her hip operation could not be performed within the foreseeable future because the hospital's budget was overspent.

The economy–efficiency–effectiveness model for evaluating health care is akin to the analytical model of health: unless it can be measured it is of no use. Against this needs to be put the holistic model of health care which takes a wider and broader view in which there are not only solutions to problems, but also aspects of care, responsibility, meaning of life and suffering, and respect for the individual.

The expansion of technology means that there are now therapies and treatments available which were never dreamt of when the NHS was conceived. But not all of these are beneficial. Neutron therapy for cancer, to take simply one example, was believed to be the most advanced form of radiotherapy and cyclotron units were purchased at vast costs. Not many years after their installation though it was found that it was worse than conventional radiotherapy for certain cancers (MacDougall et al, 1990). With the great choice of therapies and treatments available it is becoming ever more difficult to make the right or even adequate choice. With the present fall in the number of school-leavers there will not be enough nurses to care for the growing numbers of elderly people who now need more attention to stay alive and independent.

There are more worthwhile activities to be undertaken than there are human, material and organisational resources to support them. Resources put to one use will be taken away from another and the clash of priorities may be so strong that it may be impossible even to undertake some worthwhile activities (Weale, 1988).

To determine the priorities in this situation will become an ever more acute problem. The danger is that patients eventually become objects, and means to ends. Claims for excellence in the one centre are likely to become and be seen to be empire-building exercises for strong personalities, and colleagues who don't get on with each other will vie over budgets and their part in them. This has probably always been the case. With shrinking resources, more open management and certainly more public accountability there is now also more public knowledge. Perhaps economy, efficiency and effectiveness are the best values in health care? Perhaps – so long as they are tempered with ethics: the masculine model with the feminine model of receptivity, relatedness and responsivity.

Values of nursing

Many nurses say that they are not interested in politics or management but just want to get on with their job. But *how* they get on with their job is crucial. All nurses are affected by budgets, most immediately usually by shortage of staff. And all over the NHS other shortages are evident: shortage of linen, of cleaners, of security personnel or dressing packs. It is possible to make do once or twice, but when the situation becomes chronic, people lose interest and morale drops. And a dispirited nurse is not going to cheer up a patient very easily. It is less and less easy to be compassionate, committed and conscientious if all around the standards are dropping. How nurses react to such situations, not just emotionally but practically, makes them ethical nurses.

Frankl (1962) believes that the most urgent task for people is to find meaning for their lives. It could be said that nursing too has to search for its meaning, again and again. The values of society change, and with them the values of nursing change, and each generation of nurses has to discover its own values for itself. Indeed, that nursing is so sensitive to such changes is one of its strengths.

There have been debates about whether nursing is a profession, or not; about whether nursing can be independent, or not; about whether nurses can prescribe care, or not. These are all aspects of that discovery of meaning. Do nurses follow the more masculine, technical path into 'extension' by taking on more medical work like placing intravenous lines and taking blood, or do they follow the more feminine path into the 'expansion' of 'nurturing, comforting, caring, encouraging and facilitating'? (Pearson, 1983). Both aspects contain areas for care. It will depend which area will give a nurse more satisfaction in terms of being human through caring. The uniqueness of care in nursing has something to do with compassion, competence, confidence, conscience and commitment. These are some of the values which nursing is not only called to maintain, but expected by society to foster.

The values of health care are often put in terms of value for money. Decisions have to be made in the light of this and 'depending on how compassionate and civilized we want our society to be' (Salvage, 1985) we make our decisions. This may mean:

- Standing up for a personal conviction
- Defending a patient's wishes
- Pointing out inefficiencies
- Not taking 'no' for an answer
- Saying no when one means 'no'
- Getting involved when this is the right thing to do
- Defending a colleague in a difficult situation

There are no absolutely right or wrong values to hold for nurses; that would be too easy. The various values outlined in this chapter will all apply at some stage or another. One general complaint these days is always that communication is not as good as it should or could be. In the trio of receptivity, relatedness and responsiveness is enshrined the 'recipe' for good communication; without it these things would not take place. It may be appropriate, therefore, to put forward another set of values: those of communication. In dialogue there is common ground – and means to go forward. This set admirably complements the Five Cs:

- 'Be attentive
- Be intelligent

- Be reasonable
- Be responsible
- Be committed' (Johnston, 1981)

Any nurse who holds any of these values cares deeply. And by doing so is not only 'just' committed to her or his job, but is also an agent of change, a professional, a partner and a companion.

4

Ethical theories

Ethics and morality

We make many ethical decisions every day. Usually we don't think on what basis we make such decisions. Values are chosen, prized and acted upon. But ethics goes a step further, or deeper.

The word ethics comes from the Greek *ethos*, meaning character. Morals comes from the Latin word *moralis*, meaning custom, or manner. Both words mean custom, i.e. fundamental ways of conduct which are not only customary, but also right.

In popular parlance the word morality is, however, more often used for anything connected with sex or religion. Being moral implies that a person lives within a clearcut set of personal dogmas. On the other hand, ethics is more often connected with responsibility and society. Being ethical implies something cerebral, objective (Thompson, Melia and Boyd, 1983), even altruistic. Making an 'ethical investment' today means putting one's money where it is not used for arms manufacture, supporting corrupt political regimes, the tobacco industry or other unsocial aspects of one's choice. Being ethical literally means 'putting your money where your mouth is' – for those who have money. The 'investment' made by many health care workers can be just as far-reaching, and is on a far more intimate, person-to-person level.

Two approaches to ethics

There are two different ways of viewing ethics: normative and descriptive.

Normative or prescriptive ethics are to do with norms and prescriptions – the philosophical part of ethics. Philosophers down the ages have concerned themselves with how people *should* behave; they have made, or are making, the codes of conduct or ethics.

Descriptive, or scientific, ethical study has come much to the fore since the advent of the social sciences, though Socrates (469–399 BC) was condemned to death for his (too) rigorous pursuit of finding out what people thought and meant by words like 'justice' and 'virtue'. The detailed studies of sociologists, anthropologists and psychologists have given us clearer ideas of what people *actually* do than was hitherto the case, uncovering areas of personal and societal behaviour. The constraints by Victorian society on sexual matters in particular have been uncovered to a large extent by sociologists who have studied people's actual behaviour, not only what they *said* they did. Once such evidence is public, taboos about behaviour no longer need to remain taboos, and some particular behaviours pass into the area of norms. Once the majority of people think or behave in a new form, laws have to be created to accommodate this new behaviour. This in turn leads to codes which state that people *ought* or *should* behave in this way.

The difference between descriptive and normative aspects of ethics is particularly evident in health care. Doctors (traditionally men) have concerned themselves with the scientific, descriptive aspects of care. They have analysed illnesses, studied stress in relation to illness, divided people into classes and compared diseases within social classes with the aim of curing disease. This in turn has caused an explosion of high technology in medical care. Jameton (1984) asks here if the ends have justified the means. The conclusions will never be clearcut because the means of one are the ends of the other. This is the heart of ethics: goodness, justice and truth interrelate with each other, and with behaviour between people.

The normative aspects of health care have been pursued largely by nurses (traditionally women). Nurses have again and again concerned themselves with wider issues of health, such as the significance and meaning of suffering and death, and the role and purpose of caring and compassion. It is notable that in the field of care for dying people nurses have largely led the way.

Table 4.1   The two approaches to ethics

Normative(prescriptive) (what we should do)	Descriptive (what we actually do)
Mainly used by philosophers	Mainly used by sociologists, psychologists, anthropologists
Emphasis is on making recommendations for behaviour	Emphasis is on observation of behaviour
In health care:	
Pursues: • The concept of health • The significance of human suffering • Rights of patients • Dimensions of caring • Concepts, such as compassion, commitment, etc. • Meaning of death	Pursues: • Psychology of illness • Physiology of stress • Social pressures in chronic disease
Deciding whether a patient *ought* to be put on kidney dialysis	Describing *how* to put a patient on kidney machine
Traditionally the concern of nurses	Traditionally the concern of doctors

Nurses are also particularly prominent in the care of people with mental handicaps or illness.

It is important to be aware of these differences – not for the sake of argument, but for the complementarity of certain aspects, and how each can help the other in giving the best possible holistic care.

Ethical theories: two schools

Within normative ethics there are two broad, traditional schools which have shaped thinking down the ages. Their relevance to nursing is that caring has to be supplemented with competence and knowledge. A decision is only ethical if it is based on something firm. Theories supply that firm ground.

Ethical theories are complete philosophical systems in themselves, and to get to grips with them is not easy. It is only possible here to give an outline of both schools.

The ethical question in these systems is: 'What is the right thing to do?' A decision therefore depends on what is meant by 'right'. Each theory gives its answer from a different point of view.

Teleology

Teleology, or consequentialism 'defines "right" in terms of the good produced as the consequences of an action. It bids one calculate the probable results of performing various actions relevant to a situation and choose one that will maximise the ratio of benefit over harm produced' (Candee and Puka, 1984).

The best-known brand of teleology is utilitarianism. The main exponent of this theory is John Stuart Mill (1806–1873), following Jeremy Bentham (1748–1832). Mill's *Utilitarianism* was published in 1867. In it he describes the 'Greatest Happiness Principle', by saying that 'actions are right in proportion as they tend to promote happiness, wrong as they tend to produce the reverse of happiness. By happiness is intended pleasure and the absence of pain; by unhappiness, pain and the privation of pleasure.' The basic tenet of utilitarianism is 'the greatest good for the greatest number'. All actions are future-oriented; morality does not depend on any historical duty.

The difficulty with such a theory is how one can decide what is pleasure, i.e. the 'good' to be created, or what is pain and how to avoid it. To this end Mill established a theory of 'competent judges'. Only a person who has known 'higher' and 'lower' pleasures can judge truly. However, Mill forestalls such judgement by saying that the pleasures of the mind are of a higher order than those of the body. To qualify this idea, he then has to introduce a difference between quality and quantity of pleasure.

Campbell (1984b) reasons that the roots of the British welfare state lie firmly in utilitarianism. He believes that the philosophy of Mill 'lay behind reforms in conditions of employment, in the prison system, public health provision, in parliamentary representation and in the status of women'. He cites the *Report on the Sanitary Condition of the Labouring Population*, published in 1842, in which is the comment: 'It is an appalling fact that, of all born of the labouring classes in Manchester, more than fifty-seven per cent die before they attain five years of age, that is, before they can be engaged in factory labour.' The writers of the *Report* argued that the prevention of disease made economic sense; that is if people were healthy they could then work in factories. The greatest happiness therefore in this case is work and production (the 'Protestant work ethic').

Deontology

Deontology, or non-consequentialism, 'defines right by considering intrinsic features of an action, largely independent of its consequences' (Candee and Puka, 1984). In other words, the decision depends on the action itself. This theory is sceptical about an ability to look into the future and make any decisions on the consequences of actions. It therefore considers the interests and rights of a person (human rights) as of primary importance, and sees its purpose as serving the cause of justice.

The best-known advocate of this system of ethics is Immanuel Kant (1724–1804), a German metaphysician. 'For Kant, the moral problem is not how to be happy, but how to be *worthy* of happiness' (Jameton, 1984). The notion of right and wrong is also fundamental in this theory, but so is duty, or obligation. The emphasis is now not on the *action*, but on the *person*. 'A good man is one who habitually acts rightly, and a right action is one that is done from a sense of duty' (Broad, 1930). Kant has a strong sense of respect for the person and his or her capability to reason and to act morally. What or who is good or right is now judged by another, or 'higher' standard or morality. The most obvious example of such a standard is a *divine command*.

But Kant also felt that as he could not prove the existence of God, ethics and morality had to be able to stand independently, and be acceptable by all people. To this end he established a set of *moral rules* or *imperatives*.

One of these imperatives is, 'Act only according to that maxim (conventional moral rule) by which you can at the same time will that it should become a universal law' (Jameton, 1984).

This means 'that every time people are about to make a moral decision they must ask first, "what is the rule authorizing this act I am about to perform?" and, second, "can it become a universal rule for all human beings to follow?"' (Jameton, 1984). This emphasizes both the freedom of the individual, and the duty of the one for the many. A right action is only right if it is done out of a sense of duty, and the only good thing without any qualification is a person's goodwill: the will to do what one knows to be right.

Langford (1985) illustrates this by describing two nurses of equal standing and ability who work in a children's home. One works there because she enjoys this kind of work, the other because she feels that this is what she ought to be doing, even though she dislikes the children and working with them. But this second nurse has acquired a sense of civic duty. Kant therefore would judge this one as highly virtuous, and the other as someone who while doing the right thing demonstrates no moral worth as far as her work is concerned.

Kant went further and evolved the *supreme principle of morality* also called the *practical imperative*, the principle which is the highest rule: 'Treat every rational being, including yourself, always as an end and never as a mere means' (Broad, 1930). This establishes that each human being is a unique end in himself or herself, at least morally speaking.

These two theories are rarely applied to the letter now. It seems difficult to act without thinking of the consequences at all, or to act thinking only of the consequences. But as with earlier examples, it is useful to be familiar with the basic ideas of such theories because in any discussion or situation where decisions have to be made, people may start from opposing standpoints and defend one theory or the other.

Principles of ethics: 1

Ethical theories tend to be exclusive and consistent only within their own reasoning. To make them accessible one needs to have certain clear principles which embody and cover the main tenets of the theories. Jacques Thiroux (1980) has done this with a set of five principles.

Principles function like a compass: they provide the direction rather than serve as a road map. They are not rigid (as theories can be), but neither are they so flexible as to suit every whim and fancy. They will not provide the answers, but help to direct the thinking towards achieving a consensus on what ought to be done in difficult circumstances.

Thiroux's principles are applicable to any situation such as medicine, law, business, education, etc. Here they are considered in the light of nursing. In order they are the principles of:

- The value of life
- Goodness or rightness
- Justice or fairness
- Truth-telling or honesty
- Individual freedom

These principles are interdependent, but they will be described below, one after the other, for the sake of clarity.

The principle of the value of life

Thiroux sums up this principle in one phrase: 'Human beings should revere life and accept death.'

Most, if not all, known systems of morality have an injunction against killing, and for preserving life. Indeed, this is the most basic law of ethics, as 'without human life, there is no ethics'. (Some systems extend the no-killing ideal to beyond human life.)

This principle is placed first, and is held to be a near-absolute, 'because life is held both in common and uniquely by all human beings'. Life is the one thing all people have in common but each person experiences it differently. The other four principles stand, therefore, in relation to this basic one.

It does not mean that life is life 'at all costs', neither does it mean that quantity should always come before quality; indeed people *should* accept death. Thiroux argues that people should neither be killed nor have their life preserved without their informed consent, unless there is a very strong justification. (The difference between the earlier theories and these principles is the inclusion in every principle of the clause 'unless there is a very strong justification'. Ethical dilemmas only happen when there is absolutely no alternative. This is why ethical principles are not absolutes, but near-absolutes.) Because life is the basic 'given', which everybody has equally, it forms the basic premise for any discussion. A justification for taking human life is, however, there, and the following are some of the situations when life is not unquestionably either 'good' or to be preserved.

Abortion

If seen from the point of view of killing, this is an infringement of the principle of the value of life; if looked at from the point of view of the right of the person – the mother – one needs to ask: What is meant by killing, and what indeed is meant by preserving life?

Euthanasia

The advances in medical technology this century have largely created this issue. There are distinctions to be made between so-called active and passive euthanasia, and letting someone die.

Both abortion and euthanasia are discussed in more detail in Chapter 9.

Killing in self-defence

This issue qualifies the principle of the value of life in stating that one should never kill other humans except when defending innocent people, including oneself. The essence of this argument is that by threatening to kill or by killing others, killers in a sense forefeit their right to have their lives considered as valuable.

War

The idea of a 'just war' is seen to be incompatible with the reality of modern methods of warfare. War is perhaps the most powerful threat to life in general. Yet armed struggles against oppressive regimes are often the only means for nations to be heard in the outside world.

Capital punishment

It can be argued that capital punishment amounts to murder by society against one of its members. It can also be a form of societal revenge, but in a civilized society revenge should not be a valid motive for taking human life.

Suicide

This is the extreme form of self-destruction. Edel (1955) thinks that 'it is possible that ... exceptions to the value of life constitute not a *denial* of its value, but rather, an *over-balancing* of its value by other aims to which termination or deprecation of life may be instrumental'. This is clearly demonstrated by the suicide bombing of some guerrilla fighters.

Edel (1955) also asks, 'to whom is life a good?'. This question does not always have a straightforward answer. Moral dilemmas are caused because issues of good and right, justice, truth and personal freedom conflict and are valued differently. This is particularly evident when the theory of QALY (Harris, 1987) is considered. 'Quality Adjusted Life Year' is a theory developed by Professor Alan Williams in York to equate quality of life with the limited resources in health care. Simply put, the theory holds that a young medical student, critically injured, should get more treatment than a middle-aged secretary. The main criterion is life-*years* still potentially to be lived.

This theory seems to say that quantity of life matters more than quality. It is a clearly rational, money-oriented theory which has been attacked for disregarding the value of *life* and the *person's* life. Nevertheless, in a climate of economics in health care, this is a theory which may often be used openly, or more likely surreptitiously.

Nurses and carers are faced with issues of life and death every day. It is therefore important to know both one's own value-bases and also those of the person cared for. We should revere life, but also accept that it is not limitless.

The principle of goodness or rightness

This principle must *logically* be prior to the remaining principles, as the question of good and right is basic in ethics. Instead of looking at good and right in the light of consequences or rights, creating a principle of good and right combines the earlier theories now in a wider whole.

Many ethical theories are built on the assumption that everyone has, or should have, the same idea or value of good. As seen above, happiness has been described as the highest good. But other goods include life, consciousness, truth, knowledge, beauty, self-expression and so on. It is impossible to say that only one of these is intrinsically good. As society changes, so its values change, and with it what it values as good.

For an ill person, health is likely to be a good, but this concept may represent different aspects for someone with a broken nose, or multiple sclerosis. Because individuals have freedom to place more emphasis on one good or another, it does not mean that others' goods are devalued.

'Good' should not only be in the abstract, but related to other human beings. It is not possible to talk of an ethics of caring if one cannot see 'good' in relation to people – that is, in the way care is given. Thiroux argues that a sadist may gain pleasure (*his* 'good') by mistreating another human being. As this action is evidently not good, he states that 'excellence' should also be involved. Excellence makes an experience better or worse by its absence than it would be otherwise. Equally, harmony and creativity are related to good. 'If an action is creative or can aid human beings in becoming creative and, at the same time, help to bring about a harmonious integration of as many human beings as possible, then we can say it is a right action.' Kant's insistence on goodwill alludes to this sense of excellence in any action.

This principle demands:

1 That we promote goodness over badness.
2 That we cause no harm or badness.
3 That we prevent badness or harm.

This last point must be known to most nurses from Florence Nightingale's statement that hospitals should do the sick no harm. When actively doing good may not be possible, then doing no harm should be actively sustained.

The following story shows how this principle in particular can be flouted.

> Sheila was a specialist nurse in breast care. She worked with patients from two consultants. Both consultants spent time with their patients, and both told their patients that usually only a lumpectomy was necessary. When the patients saw Sheila, they told her this. However, Sheila began to notice that the patients from one consultant usually had a full mastectomy. She became alarmed and followed up one patient by going to the theatre with her. There, to her astonishment, she heard the consultant say, 'Well, that's another one duped.'

This principle means that good people should perform right actions, and that these actions should be good all the way through. This story shows that this particular consultant's actions were far from this ideal, thus jeopardizing all the other principles too.

The principle of justice or fairness

We cannot be good without being just and fair. Good people should also attempt to distribute the benefits from being good and doing right. But who should get the benefits from good human actions, and how should they be distributed?

'The moral assumptions underlying medical ethics are rarely in dispute. It is in the application of these assumptions to specific cases that the disputes arise' say Campbell and Higgs (1982). This becomes clear when certain treatments are available to some people, but not to others because of limited resources. Take kidney transplants, for example:

- Should they be available to those who deserve them, need them, or who are able in the long run to make most use of them?

The question of need is almost ruled out, as presumably everyone needs that particular treatment if they have this particular illness.

- Who decides who is to live, and how much value any person should place on his or her life?

In Britain there are far fewer patients receiving dialysis than in other European countries. On the other hand, there are many more kidney transplants than elsewhere. The distribution of scarce resources will remain an issue of justice, but:

- Do we judge according to the individual right of the person, or how much can be saved by one procedure over another?
- Does the end (saving money for other procedures) justify the means (not giving one particular treatment)?

The most ethical, just and fair way to determine who benefits from limited resources may be a fairly conducted lottery. If there are only two kidneys available, but ten people who need them, then at least a lottery would not discriminate on merit, ability, age, race or anything else. This egalitarian way seems then to be the most just in distributing good and right. In reality, the practice of drawing lots out of a hat is rare. There are rarely ten actual people waiting at exactly the same time and with the same need in any one place. It is the principle of egalitarianism which counts, but which is also so difficult to apply. It may mean that when confronted with the impossibility of upholding this principle we strive at least to do no harm.

The principle of truth-telling or honesty

As ethics takes place between and among human beings, communication is the vehicle for ethics. So that this communication can be sustained, it has to be based on truthfulness or honesty. Truth-telling is therefore fundamental to being ethical and moral.

Yet this principle is probably the most difficult one to maintain or to live. Human relationships of any kind are delicate, and to protect their own vulnerability in this area people have built up defences against exposing themselves to people. Being economical with the truth is only one way of putting this. Mark Twain apparently spoke 'as one who has told the truth a good many times in (his) life'. A quick glance at any thesaurus will reveal that in our language there are fewer synonyms for truth than for untruth or deception.

Every nurse knows how important this principle is. Unless a patient reveals clearly the symptoms which she or he is experiencing, treatment will not be accurate, and therefore not effective. But communication goes wider than facts. What is said or not said between people can drastically affect a person's mind and lead to further health or illness. The difficulty is that 'the truth' is not simply a fact, but the many perceptions around that fact which get built up with time and experience. Therefore 'the truth, the whole truth and nothing but the truth' may be a fallacy in nursing.

Henry David Thoreau said that 'it takes two to speak the truth – one to speak, and another to hear'. It is this aspect of hearing which is crucial for the telling of truth. How clients or patients perceive their truth may be more important than that we give them *our* truth.

This leads one to conclude that communication which is intended to be truly helpful may require preparation, and that therefore telling the truth is not just a matter of making a truthful statement, but of making such a statement at the right time and in the right circumstances. 'When is truth?' appears to be as relevant a question as 'what is truth?' (Mahoney, 1984).

It seems that doctors often find it particularly difficult to give patients with cancer their correct information regarding diagnosis and prognosis.

When M. L. was operated on after several months of feeling tired and nauseated, she was told that a great deal of liquid had been removed from her abdomen. She was told that she needed to rest her intestine, but that she would have some chemotherapy 'as a precaution'. She was not particularly curious about her illness, and went home to look after her mentally handicapped son, not suspecting that she had advanced carcinoma of the ovary. When she kept on vomiting she was told she had overstretched her liver; when she became breathless, that she had bronchitis. She died, unable to make any provision for her son.

Lyall (1990) reported on a survey carried out among doctors who had been asked: 'Whether they thought nurses should answer cancer patients' questions about diagnosis and prognosis truthfully.'

Ten (out of nineteen) doctors said nurses ought to evade direct questions and refer the patient to a doctor, and three felt nurses should lie to patients if they were put on the spot by a direct question. Of the remainder, four said nurses should answer if they felt able to and two said nurses could confirm that 'growth' meant cancer but should not discuss it.

This survey bodes ill for the respect doctors have of nurses' knowledge and their capacity to communicate, and for their acceptance as being equal to professional colleagues.

Benjamin and Curtis (1986) think that 'a person of integrity . . . is one whose responses to various matters are not capricious or arbitrary, but principled. One of the qualities most of us admire in others and try to cultivate in ourselves is personal integrity'.

The same authors point out that any act of deception or untruth has a corrosive effect on the relationships which are necessary to maintain social bonds. As Lyall shows, this is particularly true in nursing and medicine. It is therefore all the more surprising that both nursing and medical codes 'have traditionally been mute on the subject of truthfulness'. It seems impossible that this is just an oversight.

The principle of individual freedom

Like life, freedom is 'built into' the human structure. But freedom itself is a matter of morality; we need to use freedom to preserve life, do right and be good, act justly and tell the truth. If we had no freedom to do this, or reject it, there would be no morality. Therefore neither can this principle, nor the other four, stand alone.

As each person is unique, so each person will – and should – express the first four principles in their own unique way. This is in contrast to the earlier theories where individual freedom had no clear place. We may not be social, political, religious or economic equals, but we are all moral equals, however much some people's lifestyles differ. But moral decisions often differ because of individual differences in upbringing and life experiences.

Individual freedom is not simply something given; we need to use that freedom in order to be fully functioning individuals. The two theories outlined earlier put less emphasis on *freedom* as on the necessity to choose rightly. Freedom is not licence to do as we please, but freedom to act morally. The freedom to pick up something displayed in a shop exists, but moral freedom prevents us from stealing it.

We have freedom in the way we behave to each other and to society: how we educate our children, who we choose as friends, how we use the money earned, what books and magazines we read. Moral and ethical behaviour is seen in the consequences of any of these acts. The dilemma arises because these are *personal* acts which affect *society.* The attitude often seems to be: I choose – let the state pick up the consequences. Caring takes a different stance. It does not prescribe, or moralize; it simply points out that to care is to be human, and the human mode of being is to care. The freedom of the individual is not curtailed by this. Rather it is enhanced because the choice to care means that all other principles are also enhanced.

Principles of ethics: 2

A different set of principles of ethics is more widely known in Britain. In order, these are:

* Autonomy
* Justice
* Beneficence
* Non-maleficence

To these is often added another aspect of ethics, namely:

* Respect for the person

This set of four principles has largely been promoted by Raanan Gillon (1986), one of Britain's foremost philosophers of medical ethics. It can be argued that these principles and those of Thiroux vary little, except perhaps in language and emphasis.

The main difference is perhaps the inclusion in this present set of principles of the notion of non-maleficence. Gillon (1986) writes that: 'While it seems entirely plausible to claim that we owe non-maleficence, but not beneficence, to everybody, it does not follow from this that avoidance of doing harm (non-maleficence) takes priority over beneficence. All that follows is that the scope of non-maleficence is general, encompassing all other people, whereas the scope of beneficence is more specific, applying only to some people.'

In many instances in nursing and medicine, *non-maleficence* is certainly more applicable than *beneficence*. Treatments, operations and medications all cause 'harm' in the interest of health. If one would only consider that good (beneficence) should be done at all costs, then no one would be willing to run the risk of an anaesthetic, let alone an operation. Doing no harm is therefore an important principle because it keeps before the practitioner's mind the obligation to practise her or his skill with every respect. And this practice should cover all aspects, including that of communication. Henderson (1935) (in Duncan, Dunstan and Welbourne, 1981) writes to doctors, 'You can do harm by the process that is quaintly called telling the truth. You can do harm by lying. It will also arise from what you say and from what you fail to say. But try to do as little harm as possible.'

The difference between *autonomy* and *individual freedom* is subtle. Gillon writes of 'autonomy of action, autonomy of will and autonomy of thought'. This seems to emphasize a rather intellectual approach to the notion of freedom. Thiroux seems to have a somewhat more holistic stance when he says that, 'There are many human beings to be considered in establishing a human morality, and although they have common characteristics (bodies, minds, feelings, and so forth), each person is, nevertheless, unique.' People's needs, desires and concerns vary greatly, and to acknowledge them and accommodate them there needs to be freedom – freedom (autonomy) bounded by all the other principles.

The principle of *respect for persons* is perhaps more specific than the principle of the *value of life*. Respect for the person is rooted in the desire to avoid suffering, but precisely in doing this, it can interfere with another's freedom. The questions:

- What is a person? and
- When is someone not a person?

have been debated at great length. These issues will be taken up more specifically in Chapter 9. Suffice it here to say that paternalism (or parentalism) is seen in all its ugliness when tested against this principle.

Niebuhr's response ethics

Besides the two main and traditional theories of ethics Niebuhr's theory of responsibility is here presented as another way of expressing ethical thinking and acting. This theory is not so much an alternative as another way of expressing basic tenets. Having stressed the concept of relationship in the first three chapters, Niebuhr's theory of responsibility is a means of putting that concept into an ethical framework.

H. Richard Niebuhr (1894–1962) was an American political theologian of German extraction. He was a notable educator and leading authority on theological ethics. He was a foremost advocate of theological existentialism and together with his brother Reinhold influenced ethical thinking on both sides of the Atlantic.

Niebuhr points out that deontology asks, 'what is the law?' ('what ought I to do?'). Thus we recognize the *citizen*. Teleology asks, 'what is the goal?'. In this we recognize the *maker*. Response ethics asks, 'what is happening?', and so we recognize the *answerer*: the person who responds. This points to the basic premise that people are responsive, creative persons. All our actions are a response to actions upon us, and our interpretations of these actions. Through listening we hear (we interpret) and then we respond. We respond 'to challenge rather than from the pursuit of an ideal or from adherence to some ultimate law' (Niebuhr, 1963).

This theory has many elements of aspects outlined in earlier chapters. Niebuhr starts with the premise that to 'know thyself' is basic to all human functioning. By every activity we 'decide, choose, commit'.

This rests on a further premise: that what we have in common is our humanity. It is also a co-humanity ('Mitmenschlichkeit'): in order to stay within humanity we have to act humanly. How we interpret that humanity colours our actions. Therefore we are creative and responsive persons. This means we need freedom in order to be creative, and with fidelity to that creativity, we answer responsibly.

A creative or responsible person is one who:

- Nurtures hope
- Displays courage (as the basis of any creative relationship)
- Is committed to justice and peace
- Has a sensitivity for values which attract
- Has the capacity to admire, rejoice, contemplate
- Can value, discern and respond to the other beyond biological pressures (Häring, 1978)

Creative responsibility follows the pattern of I – Thou – We: I am aware, I listen; Thou (You) is the object of my response; We are society. In this last element is enshrined the notion of accountability. There is here a social solidarity: we respond and are responded to in a 'continuing community'.

This theory seems particularly apt for nursing. It is not abstract, like the earlier two theories could tend to be. In nursing there is a continuum of relationships, and if care is to be given at all, it depends on relationships. How these relationships function shows how we respond, how we interpret actions upon us and respond further. Both deontology and teleology tend to be coming from the masculine, isolated standpoint of 'what ought *I* to do?' and 'what is *my* aim?'. Response ethics stresses more the feminine aspect which asks 'what is happening and with whom?'. The feminine tends to look for more details and further enquiry so as to see a greater whole and more aspects of the same problem in order to respond more responsibly.

As always, both aspects are needed for any enquiry. The nursing responsibility may be to put this second, feminine aspect further to the fore at this moment so that truly holistic care *can* be given.

5

Codes and declarations

Codes

Normative, or prescriptive, ethics (see Chapter 4) is concerned with interpreting philosophical statements and theories. It is not enough to put a set of ideals before people; guidelines of ideals and theories need to be transferable into action. Codes are not laws; in a sense they come before the law. The Ten Commandments, the Hippocratic Oath, the Highway Code and the UKCC Code of Professional Conduct are all examples of such codes. They do not state or declare the obvious; they point to what should be.

Codes of practice have become more necessary in recent years. The demise of paternalistic management structures and the introduction of more public accountability demand that the accountability is based on something concrete. A code of practice is the most accessible instrument.

Main codes in nursing

The main codes for nurses practising in Britain are:

1 The International Code for Nurses.
2 The UKCC Code of Practice for the Nurse, Midwife and Health Visitor.

The first *Code of Ethics* was adopted by the International Council of Nurses (ICN) in São Paulo, Brazil, in July 1953. This Code was subsequently revised at the ICN meetings in Frankfurt,

Germany, in 1965 and again in Mexico City, in 1973 (Table 5.1).

Table 5.1 *International Council of Nurses: Code for Nurses, 1973.*
Reprinted with the permission of the International Council of Nurses

The fundamental responsibility of the nurse is fourfold: to promote health, to prevent illness, to restore health and to alleviate suffering.

The need for nursing is universal. Inherent in nursing is respect for life, dignity and the rights of man. It is unrestricted by considerations of nationality, race, creed, colour, age, sex, politics or social status.

Nurses render health services to the individual, the family and the community, and coordinate their services with those of related groups.

Nurses and people
The nurse's primary responsibility is to those people who require nursing care.

The nurse, in providing care, respects the beliefs, values and customs of the individual.

The nurse holds in confidence personal information and uses judgement in sharing this information.

Nurses and practice
The nurse carries personal responsibility for nursing practice and for maintaining competence by continual learning.

The nurse maintains the highest standard of nursing care possible within the reality of a specific situation.

The nurse uses judgement in relation to individual competence when accepting and delegating responsibilities.

The nurse when acting in a professional capacity should at all times maintain standards of personal conduct that would reflect credit upon the profession.

Nurses and society
The nurse shares with other citizens the responsibility for initiating and supporting action to meet the health and social needs of the public.

Nurses and co-workers
The nurse sustains a cooperative relationship with co-workers in nursing and other fields.

The nurse takes appropriate action to safeguard the individual when his care is endangered by a co-worker or any other person.

Table 5.1   *(continued)*

Nurses and the profession
The nurse plays the major role in determining and implementing desirable standards of nursing practice and nursing education.

The nurse is active in developing a core of professional knowledge.

The nurse, acting through the professional organization, participates in establishing and maintaining equitable social and economic working conditions in nursing.

The UKCC (United Kingdom Central Council) *Code of Professional Conduct for the Nurse, Midwife and Health Visitor* (Table 5.2) was first published in 1983 and revised in 1984. The revisions were made largely from the comments which nurses themselves had contributed, having been invited to do so in the first Code.

Table 5.2   *Code of Professional Conduct for the Nurse, Midwife and Health Visitor.* Reprinted with the permission of the UKCC.

Each registered nurse, midwife and health visitor shall act, at all times, in such a manner as to justify public trust and confidence, to uphold and enhance the good standing and reputation of the profession, to serve the interests of society, and above all to safeguard the interests of individual patients and clients.

Each registered nurse, midwife and health visitor is accountable for his or her practice, and in the exercise of professional accountability shall:

1   Act always in such a way as to promote and safeguard the wellbeing and interests of patients/clients.
2   Ensure that no action or omission on his/her part or within his/her sphere of influence is detrimental to the condition or safety of patients/clients.
3   Take every reasonable opportunity to maintain and improve professional knowledge and competence.
4   Acknowledge any limitations of competence and refuse in such cases to accept delegated functions without first having received instruction in regard to those functions and having been assessed as competent.
5   Work in a collaborative and cooperative manner with other health care professionals and recognize and respect their particular contributions within the health care team.

Table 5.2 *(continued)*

6 Take account of the customs, values and spiritual beliefs of patients/clients.

7 Make known to an appropriate person or authority any conscientious objection which may be relevant to professional practice.

8 Avoid any abuse of the privileged relationship which exists with patients/clients and of the privileged access allowed to their property, residence or workplace.

9 Respect confidential information obtained in the course of professional practice and refrain from disclosing such information without the consent of the patient/client, or a person entitled to act on his/her behalf, except where disclosure is required by law or by the order of a court or is necessary in the public interest.

10 Have regard to the environment of care and its physical, psychological and social effects on patients/clients, and also to the adequacy of resources, and make known to appropriate persons or authorities any circumstances which could place patients/clients in jeopardy or which militate against safe standards of practice.

11 Have regard to the workload of, and the pressures on, professional colleagues and subordinates and take appropriate action if these are seen to be such as to constitute abuse of the individual practitioner and/or to jeopardize safe standards of practice.

12 In the context of the individual's own knowledge, experience and sphere of authority, assist peers and subordinates to develop professional competence in accordance with their needs.

13 Refuse to accept any gift, favour or hospitality which might be interpreted as seeking to exert undue influence to obtain preferential consideration.

14 Avoid the use of professional qualifications in the promotion of commercial products in order not to compromise the independence of professional judgement on which patients/clients rely.

Applying the codes

By highlighting some of the changes made in these codes in different editions it is possible to see some of the ways in which nursing is changing.

The first *ICN Code* (1953) described the fundamental responsibility of the nurse as threefold: 'To conserve life, to alleviate suffering and to promote health.' Twenty years later (1973), this duty is seen to be fourfold: 'To promote health, to prevent illness, to restore health and to alleviate suffering.' The change must be seen in the context of the emergence of many independent countries whose health priorities were paramount, of technology to prolong life, of legislation for abortion and of rising standards of hygiene. Thus the change of the wording of a code shows also the change which is taking place in society as a whole. *Conservation of* life may not be the first priority any longer, but the word *'respect* for life' makes it now possible for nurses to challenge some life (or death) prolonging procedures.

Another interesting change is noted in the relationship with doctors. The old Code unequivocally stated that 'the nurse is under an obligation to carry out the physician's orders intelligently and loyally, and to refuse to participate in unethical procedures'. The new Code does not talk of doctors specifically, but mentions 'co-workers'. This includes all health care workers, and changes the image of the nurse as subordinate to the doctor to one of equal status and also equal responsibility with other carers.

The first significant difference between the first and second edition of the UKCC Code is in the title. The second edition is the *Code of Professional Conduct for the Nurse, Midwife and Health Visitor*, whereas the first edition was for ... *Nurses, Midwives and Health Visitors*. This, together with the use of the word 'each' in the introductory paragraph emphasizes that this code is for the *individual* practitioner.

Clause 4 was a complete addition: every nurse, midwife and health visitor should 'acknowledge any limitations of competence and refuse in such cases to accept delegated functions without first having received instruction in regard to these functions and having been assessed as competent'. This protects the nurse, but also makes her more responsible in her own work.

Clause 5 was also not present in the first edition. In bureaucracies every section of workers tends to defend its own interests. This may be useful occasionally, but on the whole it means that the receivers of care suffer when those who have another's interests at heart do not collaborate.

The clause on advertising (14) is a much clearer statement in the second edition.

Clause 11, to have 'regard to the workload of, and the pressure on, professional colleagues and subordinates' may be somewhat ambiguous. Presumably this means only nursing colleagues, as this could imply spying on the workload of *any* with whom a nurse works.

Of the two documents, the ICN Code is the more comprehensive in terms of an ethic of care. It acknowledges the universal need for nursing, the inherent respect for life and dignity and the rights of humankind. The UKCC Codes do not so much stress care, but rather the do's and don'ts of nurses if they want to remain working. Indeed, Melia (1984) believes that the UKCC Code is more useful to those who deal with cases of professional misconduct than to those who look for distinctive professional values.

The question arises:

• Can nurses use these Codes as practical bases for certain specific actions?

Following the publication of the UKCC Code, *Nursing Times* (1985a) reported the details of a case which had come before the Professional Conduct Committee of the UKCC. A staff nurse on a psychiatric unit had objected to sending a 76-year-old woman for ECT. The nurse had decided that the patient's condition contraindicated this treatment. He 'had argued that, according to the (UKCC) Code, a nurse should act in the patient's best interest'. Even though an anaesthetist had once before refused ECT as the patient was then dehydrated, and the staff nurse had discussed his decision with a senior nurse (Rea, 1985), he was dismissed for refusing to budge from his professional judgement. This nurse had believed that Clauses 1, 2 and 10 of the UKCC Code (second edition) could be relied on to back up his case, but an employment appeal tribunal upheld the dismissal from his post.

There have been numerous reports of nurses having followed the guidelines of the Code and acted as bidden. Heywood Jones (1988) documents one such case where two night sisters were so worried about the low level of staff that they had compiled a document of 130 patients in their unit, detailing: 'their problems, level of dependence and nursing requirements. This was matched to staffing allocation in order to demonstrate the inadequate and, frankly, dangerous level of cover.' This document was apparently not well received by the director of nursing services, but after an incident on that unit where a patient died due to a drug error, this document was significant. 'The admitted facts were not regarded as misconduct in view of the appalling context in which the unfortunate incident occurred. The managers were publicly criticized.' This is not the only such story. Nurses regularly use the Code as a basis for protest or drawing attention to unacceptable standards of care (Turner, 1990b).

The sad fact is that too often nurses are not heard when they complain, or are not taken seriously. When – almost inevitably – an error or accident occurs, it is the nurses who are blamed.

The Code is not meant to be a weapon with which to beat management. However, when nurses feel that they are ignored, belittled or questioned as to their motives it may be useful to defend themselves in terms of the Code. It is, after all, meant to be the basis of their professional conduct.

In a climate of strict economy and finite resources, nurses have often felt that they are not heard by the local management when they have protested about slipping standards, unacceptably low levels of staffing, or having to carry out practices for which they are not trained. In an effort to be heard, they have turned to the UKCC. This placed 'a strain on the Council's limited resources' (Swaffield, 1990b), which meant that the Council itself got accused of not reacting quickly enough.

When a nurse comes before the UKCC Professional Conduct Committee she or he will have been through several stages of investigation already. She or he may have been accused of various kinds of misconduct. In many cases this is only the visible or tangible result of failures by 'the system' which should and could have been picked up before someone got hurt.

It is to the UKCC's credit that it is 'planning more monitoring and analysis of trends and developments in professional conduct and health committee work' (Swaffield, 1990b) to put right inefficiencies in the system rather than in the nurses.

UKCC advisory documents

The UKCC has published a number of advisory documents to supplement the Code.

The first of these is a paper on *Advertising* (1985). This is a specific elaboration of Clause 14 of the Code and applies to all persons whose names appear on the professional registers. This emphasizes certain aspects of advertising of availability for work, special services, use of registration status for promotional films or literature or commercial products.

The paper *Administration of Medicines* (1986) is a lengthy document which covers prescribing and dispensing of medications, and the role of nurses, midwives and health visitors in administering medicines. It covers normal circumstances, but has, as a supplement, a section covering variations which should apply when the specified framework is not appropriate.

The Advisory Document entitled *Exercising Accountability* (1989) is 'a framework to assist nurses, midwives and health visitors to consider ethical aspects of professional practice'. According to Turner (1990b) this document helps nurses to move away from a victim role towards an assertion of nursing, and provides them with a framework and public statements about their actions. Some nurses, though, feel that *Exercising Accountability* is no more than a paper tiger which leaves nurses unaided when they need to tackle managers.

It must be understood that such documents are not rules or laws – they are guidelines, frameworks and advisory documents. It does not mean, however, that nurses can pick and choose what they like in them. If there are omissions and unworkable clauses, then nurses should take it upon themselves to have them changed. Codes can, and should, be updated and made more relevant in the light of specific cases and potential difficulties. Bergman (1976) believes that a code of ethics should not be a shield or a crutch, but 'a firm launching pad from which to project into the future'.

The subject of accountability will be dealt with in more depth in Chapter 8.

Declarations

Declarations are statements of facts, of deeds done, of actions taken. They are not laws, but are firmer documents than codes. Declarations have taken on an air of solemnity, often of urgency, and mostly contain statements of implied rights rather than of conduct. These facts are generally not disputed, but are nevertheless not easily put into practice everywhere. Among the best known such declarations are:

- The Declaration of Independence of the United States of America, written in 1776. Its second paragraph is of interest here in its choice of words and the order in which they are set: 'All men are created equal... they are endowed by their Creator with certain inalienable Rights, that among these are Life, Liberty and the pursuit of Happiness.'
- The Universal Declaration of Human Rights. Adopted by the United Nations in Paris on 10 December 1948 this Declaration has 30 articles, outlining the 'inherent dignity and the equal and inalienable rights of all members of the human family (which) is the foundation of freedom, justice and peace in the world'.

The World Medical Association has issued many declarations. These documents are binding on doctors, but are mentioned here because in certain circumstances nurses are implied because of their close cooperation with doctors. A selection of these declarations contains the *Declaration of Helsinki* (1964, revised in 1975). This contains the 'recommendations guiding medical doctors in biomedical research involving human subjects'. The *Declaration of Sydney* (1968), is a statement on the determination of death. The *Declaration of Oslo* (1970), a statement on therapeutic abortion, has as its last clause the following: 'This statement, while it is endorsed by the General Assembly of the World Medical Association, is not to be regarded as binding on any individual member association unless it is adopted by that member association' (Duncan, Dunstan and Welbourne, 1981).

The *Declaration of Tokyo* was adopted in 1975. This document contains guidelines for doctors 'concerning torture and other cruel, inhuman or degrading treatment or punishment' in relation to detention and imprisonment. Willingly or unwillingly, nurses may be in situations of assisting doctors in dubious 'research' or procedures which may be covered by this declaration.

In 1975 the International Council of Nurses issued the following resolutions related to human rights abuses (Trevelyan, 1988):

- Nurses having knowledge of physical or mental ill-treatment of detainees and prisoners take appropriate action including reporting the matter to appropriate national and/or international bodies
- Nurses participate in clinical research carried out on prisoners only if the freely given consent of the patient has been secured

after a complete explanation and understanding by the patient of the nature and risk of the research; and

- The nurse's first responsibility is towards her patients, notwithstanding considerations of national security and interest.

Declarations and codes are useful in that they provide generalized guidelines. But they have their limitations, particularly when specific issues are tested against them. The nursing codes *direct*; they do not protect; they stimulate thinking but they do not provide walls within which it is safe to act. In the overall scheme of an ethic of caring they state perhaps the obvious, or the implied, but they also sharpen the perception of care.

6

Responsibilities and rights

Responsibility

An ethic of caring is based on a basic relationship. Within this, it is based on the ability to receive through listening; to share because those concerned have been heard; and the ability to respond. For people to be and remain creative, they have to respond to people and things around them. This gives them the ability to care.

We hear a great deal these days about rights – and rightly so. But we hear much less about responsibilities. Yet the two go hand in hand.

Duty is generally linked to something prescribed or contractual. Responsibility is linked to freedom, to goodness and to rightness. Many of the words so far used (responding, responsivity, response ethic, responsibility) all link into the same thing: relating in relationships. And that is where caring happens.

Being responsible

The concept of responsibility can be divided into the more personal aspect of being responsible, and the more legal aspect of having responsibility.

Being responsible grows out of being engaged with people. It also grows out of values which come to be important as a person takes her or his stand fully in the world. Being responsible is altruistic – but it is also more than just 'doing good'. It isn't doing good on the outside to quieten a guilty conscience on the inside. It is an active taking part and interest in a cause. This may be a job, or charitable work, or local or national government. A person who feels involved is a person who is responsible.

Being responsible doesn't mean heavily bearing everybody's burdens. That would exclude the aspect of reciprocity.

To be responsible is a truly ethical act: aware of what is happening (descriptive ethics) and prepared to engage with it and work for its positive advance (normative ethics) in society.

Having responsibility

To have responsibility means to be answerable to someone or something specific, usually defined by contract. This is usually also a job for which the person is paid.

A contract lays down what the parameters of the job are, and the job-holder acts within these limits. Responsibility here means to use all one's powers to the limits, not just some of them. It means also to know the boundaries clearly and not overstep them. It would be irresponsible of a student nurse on her first placement to catheterize a patient. It would be equally irresponsible for a ward sister to see a patient with symptoms of retention and do nothing about it; or if she personally cannot act, not to use her powers of delegation correctly.

Many nurses are asked to take on extra duties in the present climate of economy. These may extend into the doctor's or into the cleaner's realms. The UKCC Code is quite specific about such situations: unless a nurse has the competence (Clause 4) she or he should not take on such duties. This is not only to safeguard herself or himself, but specifically safeguards the patient who has the right to receive care from those who are trained and educated to give that particular care. Clauses 10 and 11 (see Chapter 5) are also involved in such cases.

Rights

A person's rights are based on human needs. The state makes it a duty to protect its individual citizens by providing basic goods and services, such as clean water, food and shelter. The state also provides certain legal rights, such as the right to vote, and the right to be protected and defended. A system of policing, and criminal and civil law are in force to maintain these rights.

Generally speaking, one person's rights are another's duty. A nurse's rights are the employer's duties. A patient's rights are the nurse's duties.

A nurse's contract gives her or him the right to an established salary, paid without fail, so many days or weeks holiday, and the right to sick leave. In return her or his duty is to give care to the level of training, education and position, without fail, or that the relevant authority is informed when this cannot be done.

Nurses have the right to work in a healthy environment, free from danger of accidents to themselves or other health hazards. It is the duty of the employing authority to supply these conditions.

There are other, less clearcut, and also less obvious rights which nurses have. The institution or employing authority has a duty to promote an environment which is physically, psychologically, emotionally and spiritually healthy. In this sense nurses have a right to receive care on all levels. This essentially means that the working environment is not only healthy and safe, but also happy, conducive to work and supportive. The I and Thou of personal relationships should be echoed in an equivalent sense between employer and employee, institution and individual. A healthy environment means that an institution maintains its contracts, and has patient equipment serviced regularly and kept in good working order.

The basic duty of nurses is to care. This is seen most clearly in the relationship with patients. If patients are to be in a well-cared-for environment, then nurses have to care about that environment. This includes equipment, adequate buildings, and also relationships with co-workers.

The relationship with employers is not always easy as it is mostly one of duty, and often one of suspicion and calculated friendliness. In a study on burnout in nurses Albrecht (1982) found that the least burntout nurses were those who were involved in the hospital environment through support groups, discussions with their supervisors, and those who were keen to be in on policy formation for their various work-units. The duty to care well for patients may, therefore, have the wider aspect of caring also for the environment of care.

An institution's rights and duties

The nurses' rights are the institution's duties. An institution has wide duties to many groups of employees.

A hospital or health authority as an institution has first of all a duty to care for its patients. It takes this from the state who sees health care for all as its duty, and as the individual citizen's right. As such it is merely carrying out its legal responsibility.

But ethics are above law, and a good action is only good if there is a sense of 'excellence' attached to it.

An institution, therefore, that acts ethically acts in such a way that it prevents, foresees, actualizes potential and humanizes. It creates a caring environment. It sees its duties not only as strictly 'having to', but more as 'wanting to'. This is often evident in the atmosphere in an institution. Where there is care, there is less stress, people are relaxed and aware of a sense of wellbeing. When the staff is well cared for and respected, the patients are more likely to be treated in the same way.

An institution, whether hospital, health authority or management team of any description, has a duty to maintain high standards of patient care, and do this actively, by promoting and legislating policies that will ensure this. Simply to maintain the status quo is not adequate, as constant changes ask for constant reappraisal and realignment of policies and byelaws.

The rights of an institution are that it can expect its employees to respect such policies and measures, and help others to respect them.

An inherent difficulty in these matters is due to the fact that an institution is made up of individuals, and their own rights and obligations may conflict with those of the institution. The language of rights tends to emphasize negative rights – in other words, the protection of what we have, and not the positive rights, or the provision of what we need. The patient has a right not to come to harm in hospital, but he also has the right to receive care which actually helps him to get better.

Individual and collective rights and duties conflict often because what an individual needs – such as health care – cannot be provided by the collective membership. The concept of advocacy arose out of such situations.

The ethical principles mostly involved here are those of justice and fairness, and non-maleficence (see Chapter 4). But it is difficult to say that one aspect of ethics is more important than another, because if one principle is compromised, all the others are too. Justice in health care is more and more an issue of concern because as more care is available, more will be needed, but the purse is not tied to an endless supply of money.

The patient's rights

Britain's Patient's Charter is still under discussion (1992). The American Hospital Association published its Patient's Bill of Rights in 1973. Set in a system of government with a constitution, and patients mostly paying for their health care, this Bill is not equally applicable in the UK. It is nevertheless printed here, but for reference and interest only (Table 6.1).

Table 6.1   *A Patient's Bill of Rights: American Hospital Association, 1973.* Reprinted with permission of the American Hospital Assocation, copyright 1972

---

1   The patient has the right to considerate and respectful care.
2   The patient has the right to obtain from his physician complete current information concerning his diagnosis, treatment and prognosis in terms the patient can be reasonably expected to understand. When it is not medically advisable to give such information to the patient, the information should be made available to an appropriate person on his behalf. He has the right to know, by name, the physician responsible for coordinating his care.
3   The patient has the right to receive from his physician information necessary to give informed consent prior to the start of any procedure and/or treatment. Except in emergencies, such information for informed consent should include, but not necessarily be limited to, the specific procedure and/or treatment, the medically significant risks involved, and the probable duration of incapacitation. Where medically significant alternatives for care or treatment exist, or when the patient requests information concerning medical alternatives, the patient has the right to such information. The patient also has the right to know the name of the person responsible for the procedures and/or treatment.

Table 6.1 *(continued)*

4 The patient has the right to refuse treatment to the extent permitted by law, and to be informed of the medical consequences of his action.

5 The patient has the right to every consideration of his privacy concerning his own medical care program. Case discussion, consultation, examination and treatment are confidential and should be conducted discreetly. Those not directly involved in his care must have the permission of the patient to be present.

6 The patient has the right to expect that all communications and records pertaining to his care should be treated as confidential.

7 The patient has the right to expect that within its capacity a hospital must make reasonable response to the request of a patient for services. The hospital must provide evaluation, service and/or referral as indicated by the urgency of the case. When medically permissible a patient may be transferred to another facility only after he has received complete information and explanation concerning the need for, and alternatives to, such a transfer. The institution to which the patient is to be transferred must first have accepted the patient for transfer.

8 The patient has the right to obtain information as to any relationship of his hospital to other health care and educational institutions insofar as his care is concerned. The patient has the right to obtain information as to the existence of any professional relationships among individuals, by name, who are treating him.

9 The patient has the right to be advised if the hospital proposes to engage in or perform human experimentation affecting his care or treatment. The patient has the right to refuse to participate in such research projects.

10 The patient has the right to expect reasonable continuity of care. He has the right to know in advance what appointment times and physicians are available and where. The patient has the right to expect that the hospital will provide a mechanism whereby he is informed by his physician or a delegate of the physician of the patient's continuing health care requirement following discharge.

11 The patient has the right to examine and receive an explanation of his bill regardless of source of payment.

12 The patient has the right to know what hospital rules and regulations apply to his conduct as a patient.

Davis and Aroskar (1983) say that this document is well-intended, but timid. They believe that since these rights were invested in the patient to begin with, the hospital has no power to grant these rights. Indeed, it seems pretentious to return rights – and with an air of largesse – which the hospital previously stole from the patients. Perhaps it should therefore be termed 'A Hospital's Bill of Duties'?

The Bill outlines some basic facts: that the 'healing process' is a matter of cooperation; that the relationship between patient and physician is crucial to this cooperation, and based on trust; and that the patient has the last word. Thus paternalism in health care is seen to be not only unhelpful, but positively unethical.

The patient's (British and American) rights are the human rights of individuals: the freedom to choose; the right to knowledge and dignity; and the right to self-determination. But a patient also has certain duties. For a diagnosis to be established, a patient needs to disclose all relevant information fully and frankly. The exchanges between doctor and patient depend on this duty, for unless truth is told, truth cannot be told in return. The same principles of course apply to communication between patient and nurse.

Responsibilities and rights in action

The following story will highlight certain concepts just outlined:

> Don, an elderly, rather heavy gentleman, was in hospital following a stroke which left him paralysed on his left side. He was transported to the bath every day sitting on a hoist. One particular day the nurse who was allocated to care for him had noticed that the handle of the hoist was not turning properly. Just outside the bathroom the seat of the hoist became loose and fell away from the stem. Don's paralysed leg was trapped underneath the seat and himself, breaking in three places.

The patient's rights can be listed as:

- To adequate (careful) care.
- To be respected as a person.
- To leave hospital as quickly as possible in a better state than when entering.
- To come to no harm from buildings, equipment or inadequate care.

The nurse's duties will include some of the following:

- To give adequate (careful) care.
- Not to use defective equipment but to report it for repair.
- To use her education and experience adequately.
- Not to take risks.
- Not to harm the patient.

Her responsibilities will be all those above, and additionally:

- To be responsible for her action.
- To have due regard for the environment of care (UKCC Code Clause 10) and if necessary do something about it before it is too late.
- To give a good example by her actions – or conversely, not to let standards slip by conforming to pressures.
- Not to bring the profession into disrepute by her actions.

Many responsibilities and duties are only seen clearly when something has gone wrong. Values are only discovered through challenges. When an accident or suffering forces a person to search for the sense and the meaning of it, then only does it become clear.

The UKCC Code is essentially a document of what a nurse's responsibilities are. The way in which these are interpreted does, however, depend on the individual. The Code is not a stick, nor are responsibilities heavy burdens. As usual, there is a balance to be achieved between both of them.

Responsibility is not complete without accountability. As this has become a major issue in nursing it will be dealt with specifically in Chapter 8.

Since this text was written the British Government has published its Patient's Charter, and this should now be set alongside the Patient's Bill of Rights quoted in this chapter.

7

Making ethical decisions

Making choices

It has been said that nurses find it easier to talk of making sensible or successful decisions rather than making ethical decisions. Perhaps the reason for that is that they don't know what ethical issues are, and consequently don't know how to make ethical decisions. Hopefully, this book will help with both these issues.

Before a decision can be made, there has to be a choice. At least two alternatives need to be available. They may not always be very clearcut. But so that eventually a decision can be made all the possibilities and alternatives have to be seen and recognized. Mayeroff (1972) says that if we want to care, we need to know many things (see Chapter 1). Nevertheless, many ethical decisions are made without much probing or deliberating. Some people believe that these are the best decisions. Others think the opposite, and believe 'that the longer a decision takes and the choices are weighed, the greater the efficiency' (Sigman, 1979).

Nurses are often in situations where decisions have to be made quickly. It is only after the event that they realize that these were deeply ethical decisions.

But there are also situations where much deliberation has to take place. An ethical decision is never made 'cold', on paper; it always concerns people. The following is such an example.

Doreen was the ward sister of a medical oncology ward. She became suspicious when she noticed that the consultant always spent more time on his rounds with some patients than with others, and prescribed more elaborate treatments for some than for others. Doreen guessed that the consultant asked these patients for payments, but she had no way of finding out. She could not discuss her suspicions with anybody because if she did and she was wrong, then the consultant could make her life very difficult. If she was right, then the consultant's life would be made difficult. She kept her eyes and ears open. One day a patient made a remark which confirmed her suspicions. From then on, Doreen recorded her findings. A whole year later she had made her decision: she left to take up an art course, and at the same time told her story to a newspaper. As a result the consultant was arrested and imprisoned not only for professional misconduct, but also for not declaring taxes.

This incident took place in a country with a system similar to the NHS. Doreen was in a difficult position. Her sense of right and wrong led her to decide that it was wrong to abuse the health system facilities, and to extort patients. But if she talked, a scandal might be created from which no one benefited, and no action might follow. She had to be sure of her facts, and also how she could strike a decisive blow. In the end, she sacrificed her nursing career, but her action uncovered many other wrong dealings in high places.

In this sense, Doreen followed the consequentialist model (see Chapter 3); she thought through what would be the consequences of her actions both for herself and for the consultant, and she acted accordingly.

A non-consequentialist might say that the act of exposing wrongdoings itself is good, regardless of the consequences to the people involved.

How then, are ethical decisions reached? Nurses are familiar with the four steps of the nursing process for arriving at solving problems. In making ethical decisions the four steps of assessing, planning, implementing and evaluating are equally valid. Several models (Aroskar, 1980a; Jameton, 1984; Crisham, in Scott, 1985)

Table 7.1 Models for ethical decision-making

Jameton's model	*Crisham's model*		*Nursing process model*
Identify the problem	M	'Massage' the dilemma	Assessment
Gather data			
Identify options	O	Outline options	
Think the ethical problem through	R	Review criteria/ resolution	Planning
Make a decision			
Act	A	Act	Implementation
Assess	L	Look back/ evaluate	Evaluation

have been developed, all more or less along the lines of the decision-making process (Table 7.1). Seedhouse (1988) has developed an 'ethical grid' which is interesting but too lengthy to describe in detail here.

The basic model of problem-solving is used here and elaborated with a series of questions. They are by no means all the questions which could be asked, but they can stimulate further questions and different probing. The problem-solving approach is rather 'masculine', linear, and even rigid. An ethic of caring will want to pay particular attention to the 'feminine' aspects of more circular or spiral thinking and acting. Questions which come from this quadrant are, therefore, specifically emphasized. This does not mean that these questions are particularly important. They simply point out aspects which may have been neglected and which nurses are in a leading position to advocate. In a decision-making situation it is crucially important to recognize all aspects, otherwise a decision can never be said to have been well made. Masculine and feminine emphases should therefore both be available and used.

Step One: Assessment

Often enough a problem is never stated clearly. Or if more than one person is concerned, assumptions are made by both parties that they know what is going on. But each side comes from a different background, and this will mean different perceptions and different values. Or again, a problem is seen generally, not in detail. 'The care in this district is not good enough' has to be made very specific before it can be changed. Stating the problem in terms of people is perhaps the most realistic as eventually choices and outcomes directly affect people: you and me.

The first step asks Niebuhr's question: 'What is happening?' In an ethic of caring this must always be the question of most concern. This is not just curiosity; it shows genuine empathy and a willingness to 'be there', to receive, to share, and to respond with all the compassion, competence, confidence, conscience and commitment possible.

This first step asks, assesses and analyses. It clarifies details, seeing everything in terms of facts:

- Is it an actual or a potential problem?
- What is the history of the problem?
- Why is it a problem which cannot be solved easily?
- Which facts are important? Which facts are irrelevant or unimportant?
- Are there any aspects which enhance or go against the conscience of any person involved?
- Who are the people directly involved?
- What is the role of each involved person?
- How does each person perceive the problem?
- Who are the key people?
- What are the key people's overall nursing, medical and social situations?
- Are there aspects which can be changed or which cannot be changed?
- How is this problem like or unlike other situations or similar cases?
- What other relevant considerations are there?
- Is the futility of further treatment questioned?
- Is it a question of opposing values?
- Which ones are more important? Why?

- Is it a question of professional relationships?
- Is any clause in the code of professional conduct invoked?
- Is there a clear duty involved for anyone?
- Does this change or influence the situation?
- What are the basic (human) needs involved?
- What are the wants and desires of the individuals?
- How do the needs and wants compare?

The principles will help to state the problem in terms of ethics:

- Does the problem encroach on the principle of the value of life, i.e. is it a question of shortening or prolonging life, questioning the quality of life or the sanctity of life?
- What is good or right about the situation; what is not good or right? People are seen to be good and actions right: who is good or not good; what is right, or not right?
- Is it a problem which should be seen in terms of justice? What is questioned about justice?
- Is it a problem of truth-telling or honesty – or lack or disregard of it?
- Is it a problem of individual freedom or autonomy?
  How does the problem encroach on this principle?
- Are all persons respected equally?

When all the fact-finding questions have been asked, what is left is the need for care. Some of the questions which relate specifically to care are:

- Has everybody been heard, and have they said all they needed to say?
- How have relationships been affected by this problem?
- Which are the significant relationships involved?
- What does the 'significant other' say, feel, convey, or wish to happen?
- How does that affect the other relationships?
- Who has suffered, and in what way, so far?
- What are the main feelings expressed by the various parties? What do they indicate, or point to?
- How has care been affected so far?

An ethic of caring will endeavour to see as many points as possible. This will include in particular the feelings which people are aware of, as these are the basis for any meaningful outcome.

Step Two: Planning

Step Two, the planning stage asks that the now clarified problem be looked at in terms of how care is best given and an ethics of care is best served.

At this stage it becomes obvious which theory a person is to follow:

- Is it a question of deontology, i.e. what ought to be done? The action itself counts?
  or
- Is it a question of teleology, i.e. of the outcome of an action? The consequences matter?
- Is it a question of response ethics, i.e. responding to the individual, and how all protagonists can be most creative, responsive persons in, through, and beyond this situation?

The first two questions may overlap, as any action has outcomes and consequences. But the emphasis may differ. The third question is in a different category, but essentially includes the first two.

This step is concerned with the future, therefore all the questions are future-oriented. Some questions relevant to this step may be:

- What actions are possible?
- What are short-term or long-term possibilities?
- What are the possible outcomes of each action?
- Who will be helped in particular?
- How likely is any one outcome?
- Will anybody be hurt by any particular outcome? If so, how?
- Will one decision solve the problem, or are there likely to be further decisions to be taken?
- Is there a time limit?

According to Jameton (1984), this is the point when ethical theories will now have to be thought through, and the problem tested against them.

- In what respect does the principle of the value of life give direction at this stage? The summary of that principle is: 'Human beings should revere life and accept death'. In what way should life be revered here (if it is not) or death accepted (if it is not)? Is there an action which has to be taken to uphold this principle, an outcome to be hoped for, or ways looked for by which all involved can be more creative persons?
- In which way are good or right compromised? Can all persons involved be 'good', i.e. act according to values and principles, enhance the common good, keep and enhance integrity, creativity and any other human characteristics which increase rather than decrease personal and societal wellbeing?
- How are any specifically-planned actions right or wrong for any individual, all concerned in the situation and/or the wider context? Will an action affect one or many people, and is that as it should be? How could an action be made more right, more specific and with better consequences?
- What aspects of justice or fairness are involved? (The emphasis here is on distributive justice or equity, not legal justice.) How is justice served by this action? How might justice be harmed by this action? For a person to be good, she or he needs not only to be free, creative, respectful of others in *thought*, but in action. How can justice be seen to be done?
- How is the principle of truth-telling or honesty involved? Can all speak the truth freely? Do all of them speak the truth freely? Truth-telling enhances relationships: how are the present relationships enhanced by truth? In relationships people become creative and responsive: in what way does truth help them in this fundamental quest to be and become authentic human beings? Is the act of telling the truth itself right, or what would the consequences be if it were, or were not told?
- Individual freedom and autonomy are the elements which make human beings unique. Is this principle upheld, or not, by this action? Is there any coercion around anywhere? Who gives freedom to whom? Who or what takes freedom from whom or from what?
- Is harm being caused? How can it be minimized?
- Is the general tone of the discussion or search for solution respectful and conducive to good and right above the merely necessary?

The ethical grid which Seedhouse (1988) developed is more clearly divided into deontological (duty ethics) and teleological (consequentialism) aspects. According to this latter, some of the questions to be asked should therefore be: Does the proposed action or intervention bring:

- An increase of individual good.
- An increase of self-good.
- An increase of the good of a particular group.
- An increase of social good?

When ethical choices have to be made they are often seen in terms of one or all, the individual or the group, the self or society. When a situation is truly seen ethically it is evident that it is never a question of a clear either/or. The individual influences society; society influences the individual.

The specifically caring side of ethics has one very important question at this step:

- What is the meaning of it?

Frankl (1962) was very clear that people who have or followed a meaning are people with a purpose. They strive towards a goal. By doing this their actions are purposeful and are subject to that goal. While it is clearly possible to pursue a goal which is not conducive to the common good, it must be evident that an ethic of caring is an ethic with a positive aim. Every ethical decision has a consequence, and people have to live with it. If this consequence can be seen not in terms of grinning and bearing it, but in terms of creativity, then the meaning of it has to be discovered, somehow. This may not always be evident, and indeed if it isn't, the prior question may have to be:

- Is there a potential for meaning in this situation?

A commitment to caring does imply also a commitment to the potential for creativity and caring in a person.

An ethic of caring will want to be free – and is free – to explore also the unusual and the unexpected. The hallmark of such an ethic is its creativity and potential for responding to creativity. This will often include clearly imaginative thinking, lateral thinking, including transcendental aspects and insights. These help to shape the meaning of life and the changes in people's lives. It is, therefore, important that these features are acknowledged, heard, included in discussions and acted upon appropriately.

The other equally important element to consider is the specific relationship of any one person with the patient or client. This is far from always the most obvious person. Grandchildren, lovers and neighbours may all have a special claim. Often it may also be a particular nurse, doctor, or other health care personnel. And not to be forgotten are pets. They cannot answer to care, but many people's lives are entirely centred round them, and this needs to be acknowledged in the most imaginative way possible.

When the many and varied aspects of the choice in a situation have been gone over carefully, an end may be in sight.

- Is a consensus emerging?
- If not, who would have to make a decision?

At this stage it may become clear that more issues are involved than were at first evident. If this is the case, and they conflict, it may be better to look at them separately and go through the various processes again with each one.

Conversely, having studied the problem so far, it may become clear how to solve it. The example of Doreen shows that her action followed a line of logical thinking and preparation. The problem may even turn out to be easier to solve than was at first thought!

Step Three: Implementation

To decide ethically is the moral ability; to act ethically is the physical ability. Decisions do not only have to be taken, they also have to be carried out. If the decision, for instance, was to turn the machine off, then it has to be done. But there is more to the act than mechanically turning a switch. Even this can, and should, be done in a caring way. The most appropriate person should do it in the most appropriate way.

Every caring act is an ethical act. Every nurse can give an injection, but *how* the injection is given counts.

One of the criteria against which one acts must surely be:

- Would I like to be treated in this way?

Step Four: Evaluation

Evaluation of any action is crucial, but rarely easy.

If the decision was that active treatment should be stopped for a dying person, then presumably the person will die. How the death took place, and how the family reacted may then be taken as an evaluation.

If at birth it was decided to treat a severely handicapped baby, then an evaluation may really only be made years later when the quality of life of that person and of the parents, will be evident.

Between these two extremes lie a host of other situations which will be having less obvious outcomes, but nonetheless important ones. The most difficult situations are always relationships. How they are upheld, mended, ended or lived with are practical outcomes of decisions which involved choices based on values and principles. One situation may guide a person to make a particular decision expecting a similar outcome.

The people who have gone through the decision-making process together should ideally also be together for an evaluation session. This may of course not always be possible. Some of the questions which may help an evaluation might be:

- Has the decision solved the problem? If not, why not?
- In what way has the solution of one particular problem affected the wider issue?
- Were the expected outcomes realistic? If not, why were they not realistic?
- Were only particular aspects realistic? Which ones were they?
- Why were some aspects not realistic?
- If you had to decide again, would you decide in the same way? If not, why not?
- Has a greater good been achieved?
- Have other people also benefited by the original decision?
- Have further similar decisions been easier to make because of this one?
- Has any aspect of this ethical decision now become a universal law?

The importance of evaluation of ethical problems cannot be overstated. In nursing there is a tendency to bumble from crisis to crisis without learning much from each one. When it is possible to learn from one problem, the next *problem* may not be easier, but the *process* for solving it may save everyone involved both mental and physical energy.

An ethic of caring will always look to the future, the greater, the whole picture, the person's whole life. Thus an evaluation will be seen in this wider context.

- What has been gained by this decision?
- (How) is the person now 'more' a person?
- How can this help others in similar situations?
- What about the people with significant relationships to the patient or client; how do they now feel, or cope? What has changed for them? What meaning is there now for them in what has happened?
- Have any earlier fears been allayed?
- What of all the feelings expressed – how have they changed, and to what?

These are only some possible questions to guide someone in the direction of ethical thinking. In most situations such questions are at best theoretical because the situation cannot be fitted to the questions. Those involved in any decision-making process have to approach each situation afresh. This is perhaps the challenge of ethics.

8

Ethical issues in nursing

Ethical issues

Most of the ethical issues in nursing are problems of constraints:

> The hospital nurse finds herself constrained in various and
> occasionally conflicting ways by the hospital (which employs
> her), the physician (with whom she works), the client (for
> whom she provides care), and the nursing profession (to
> which she belongs). To what extent can she be her own
> person – i.e. be ethically autonomous – in these circum-
> stances? (Benjamin and Curtis, 1986).

This is a very neat division of the many ethical issues which
nurses face every day.

But such a division is never quite so easy in practice. In fact,
Campbell and Higgs (1982) show that in most incidences all
disciplines and layers are involved. They also show how easy it
is to overlook the real problem: everyone is so busy making the
right decision for themselves that the patient is never heard.

> If we cannot produce solutions, it is always important to be
> able to offer enough time to listen to the person and hear
> what is to be told. We cannot ever close the divide between
> ourselves and others: but we can pay attention to what they
> tell us they see on their side.

It is this last point which is stressed again and again as being the caring stance.

In looking at some of the many ethical issues which are regularly around in nursing under various clear headings, it must be stressed that each issue could also be dealt with just as well under another heading. The overlap does not make the issue easier. It simply makes it more imperative for the nurse to be aware that making ethical choices involves 'individuality, being awake to responsibility (and) a willingness to make personal choices' (Niblett, 1963).

Ethical issues between nurses and patients

Many issues of ethical importance in the relationship between nurses and patients have already been touched on. They are mainly to do with the type of care given. The Five Cs (see Chapter 1) define care in terms of values. These set the stage for actions which are ethically right. In this section, therefore, only a few specific issues will be considered more clearly.

Confidentiality

All nursing codes of ethics (see Chapter 5) have a clause regarding confidentiality. The question is:

- What is meant by confidentiality?
- What is confidential material?

Baly (1984) writes of legal and moral aspects of confidentiality.

The legal sides of confidentiality concern particularly the patients' case notes. The Data Protection Act (1984) protects computerized records, but does not cover any manually recorded documents. Vast numbers of people have regular or casual access to case notes, and these have an uncanny habit of getting lost. As long as they are written by hand or typewriter they are not protected at present, and their 'loss' could be potentially dangerous.

The RCN (1980) *Guidelines on Confidentiality in Nursing* makes a distinction between giving information to a court of law, or the police. In a court of law all information must be given, but to the police only such information as is 'sufficiently in the public interest to be justifiable'. For disclosure of other information the advice of an authority – such as a hospital administration – should be sought.

The UKCC advisory paper on *Confidentiality* (1987) lists four categories under which information may be disclosed:

(a) With the consent of the patient/client.
(b) Without the consent of the patient/client when the disclosure is required by law or order of a court.
(c) By accident.
(d) Without the consent of the patient/client when the disclosure is considered necessary in the public interest.

Moore (1988) believes that category (d) will present most difficulty to nurses. This aspect relates to such matters as serious crime, child abuse and drug trafficking. But what precisely constitutes a 'serious crime' is difficult to decide for a nurse. On the other hand, problems of child abuse and alcohol and substance abuse are more often encountered by nurses.

> Carrie was a health visitor on a suburban housing estate. When she visited a mother and her baby, the 15-year-old daughter of her husband's previous marriage proudly proclaimed that she could name a mate in each of the blocks who was using drugs.

● How does a nurse combine confidentiality and safeguarding the lives of fellow citizens?

The UKCC advisory paper urges practitioners always to discuss any matter fully with other practitioners (not only or necessarily fellow nurses, midwives or health visitors). Whoever holds confidential information has to be very careful not to divulge it without due consideration. The UKCC advisory paper states that:

> the responsibility to either disclose or withhold confidential information in the public interest lies with the individual practitioner, that he/she cannot delegate the decision, and that he/she cannot be required by a superior to disclose or withhold information against his/her will.

On matters relating to treatment, or the patient's illness, discussion and disclosure may, or even must, take place. 'Disclosure to a doctor might be, and probably would be, privileged and would not put the nurse under any legal liability,' says the RCN document. The condition of privilege, meaning a right, immunity or special advantage, applies to persons and information concerned with a patient or client, but 'privilege would be lost if the information was known to be malicious or damaging' (Baly, 1984).

Nurses will hear many a tale in the course of duty. Sometimes this may present the missing link in a person's story and may be most helpful in the care to be given. Some such nuggets often turn up unexpectedly, with a patient adding, 'but didn't you know?'. At other times, confidences are made simply because there is a special relationship between nurse and patient. One such case is the patient who had recently remarried after a divorce twice before, but his present wife was only aware of one previous marriage. Knowing this would not have changed his care, the nurse kept the information to herself. But in the point made above, all those involved may gain by knowing more about a patient.

A good rule of thumb here may be: when in doubt ask the patient or client. Would she or he be happy to have the information disclosed? Most information given to professionals is not a secret, but rather than presume, it is not only polite but also truly respectful of the person, to ask if what they had revealed can be passed on to the relevant authority so that he or she can be helped more effectively. This may sound contradictory when it concerns a crime or abuse. But the need is first of all to help, only second to punish.

Since 1 November 1990 patients have the unqualified right of access to information in manually-held health records, through the Access to Health Records Act (1990). Access to computerized records is restricted to patients though under certain conditions these can be made available (Tingle, 1990a).

Confidentiality is a complex issue which is too easily overlooked and too often breached. It is an issue over which nurses are often in conflict with doctors. Nurses don't have to be spies, but be on their guard that patients' rights are not infringed or taken for granted. If they are, nurses truly become advocates.

Advocacy

Curtin (1979) bases a philosophy of nursing on the concept of advocacy. She says that an advocate is first and foremost a person who can and does enter into a relationship with another person. Advocacy is based upon our common humanity, our common needs, and our common human rights.

Advocacy is not something straightforward, and neither is it something that should get the 'tomato sauce' treatment, i.e. 'labelling almost anything as advocacy and believing it can be added to anything, even very traditional practice, and somehow it will be enhanced' (Wolfsenberger 1977, in Thomason, 1987).

It may be useful to look at advocacy both from the positive and negative side, that is why it should be practised, and why it should not be practised.

Why advocacy should be practised

An advocate is one who pleads the cause of another. To do that, the advocate needs to know a great many things about the person on whose behalf she or he pleads, and also about the reasons why the patient or client needs pleading for. The advocate has to have a good understanding of the 'common humanity' which largely corresponds to the 'reciprocity' of earlier chapters. She or he has to know the patient's needs, and that means a receptivity which can only come from listening and hearing and an empathy which goes beyond simply the superficial wants of either party involved. And third the advocate needs to know the human rights involved, and that points to the 'responsivity' mentioned so often already. To know the rights and see the needs is one thing; to do something – to respond in a caring and ethical way – is quite another. There needs to be courage which is born of compassion, otherwise all talk of advocacy is simply window-dressing. Advocacy is, therefore, a fundamental aspect of an ethic of caring.

Curtin (1979), quoting Nietzsche, says that 'he who has the why to live can bear with almost any how', and goes on to say that 'we must – as human advocates – assist patients to find meaning or purpose in their living or in their dying'. The concept of advocacy above all others embodies the ideals of an ethic of caring: listening; the relationship between I and Thou; and acting with compassion, competence, confidence, conscience and commitment.

According to Brown (1985) there are four reasons why nurses should advocate on behalf of patients. These areas largely correspond to the five principles of ethics (see Chapter 4). The first area for advocacy is the quality of care which a patient receives (corresponding to the principles of the value of life, and of goodness or rightness). The second area involves the access to care by the patient (the principle of justice or fairness). Third, the patient should be fully informed about the care which he receives – that is, he should have reasons, effects and side-effects explained and understand them (the principle of truth-telling or honesty). Finally, a patient should understand the alternatives to the care proposed (the principle of individual freedom).

These various aspects of advocacy make it clear that ideally the patients or clients should:

> have enough information to enable them to exercise control over their own health care, that their legal and moral rights are respected and that health care resources are adequate to provide an appropriate quality and quantity of care (Webb, 1987).

Thomason (1987) describes four different levels of advocacy:

- A personal level – such as the help provided by many voluntary groups to individuals.
- A professional level – advocacy provided by solicitors and others.
- A public level – where campaigns take place, demanding better services.
- A practical level – advocacy as innovation, demonstrating new projects and being catalysts for new services.

A new concept in this field is 'citizen advocacy' whereby ordinary people establish a 'one-to-one relationship with vulnerable individuals, acting on their behalf to identify needs, represent interests and stand up for their rights' (Thomason, 1987).

Most of the argument for advocacy is that under normal circumstances a patient or client should have enough 'how' to advocate for himself or herself and so find, or pursue the 'why' of his or her life.

Why advocacy should not be practised

Walsh (1985) argues that nurses will not make effective patient advocates because while they are employed by the institution in which a patient is, they will always be concerned about their own job or career, or the need of the employer. The relationship of advocate with patient would in this way be compromised.

A similar stance is taken by Porter (1988) whose argument is based on the American sociologist Talcott Parsons. Parsons had described the 'sick role' of a person in a health care system which had become a social structure which in itself causes disease. Those who are part of that system assist each other to maintain that social order of health and illness and therefore have a vested interest in maintaining power as professionals. Advocacy, maintains Porter, can in this instance at best be a kind of 'benign paternalism'.

Brown (1986), a student nurse when writing, believes that being an advocate remains an optimistic and ideal portrayal of what nurses do.

> Those who want to be patient's advocate at all are rarely in a position where they can be effective as such: they are either junior nurses, who have little or no contact with doctors or treatment decisions anyway, or they are nurse academics, not involved in day-to-day patient care.

This seems to be borne out in a survey by Gramelspacher et al (1986) carried out in a university hospital. Fifty doctors and nurses were asked to say what they considered to be ethical problems. Not considering what these are here, only:

> fifteen of the subjects said that they recognized ethical problems daily, and a further twenty-nine thought that they encountered ethical problems at least once a month. The remaining three nurses and three doctors perceived such problems as infrequently as once every six months.

If nurses and doctors are so unaware of ethical problems, how can they be advocates? What would they be advocating about?

Nurses often see advocacy in terms of 'fighting the system'. Brown (1986) makes the point that if 'the system' were good, patients would not need advocates. By implying that they do, we are only 'shoring up an iniquitous system'. Indeed, by identifying with 'the depressed, angry, frustrated and unhealthy patients' nurses use patients as an 'excuse for being miserable'. This is saying that nurses do not have the courage to stand up for themselves and change their outlook and behaviour because they are afraid of what might happen if they do. It is, therefore, easier to project inadequacies and frustrations on the helpless patients. It makes one feel better that way, and one may be deemed as 'good' by others. But this, according to Brown, only makes nurses 'parasites on another's weakness'. She calls on nurses to rid themselves of insecurities which make them suspicious and defensive towards patients who know 'too much' or show an interest in their treatment.

- Can or should the nurse give the patients more information?
- Does the patient have the right to receive from the nurse information withheld by other professionals?
- To whom is the nurse responsible: the patient, the doctor or her conscience?
- How can a nurse be an effective advocate in situations of conflict?

The issue of advocacy is certainly not easy. It crosses into several areas of responsibility. Self-advocacy may sound like an excuse for getting involved; perhaps the most effective way of caring ethically is empowering others. 'Advocacy is a means of transferring power back to the patient to enable him to control his own affairs' (Brown, 1985). As in so many other areas of care, the key seems to lie in the relationship between carer and cared-for. The carer who can look at facts and feelings, at masculine and feminine ways of perceiving a situation – that carer knows when and how to be an advocate – or not.

Ethical issues between nurses and doctors

The relationship between nurses and doctors is a particularly important one. It is a working relationship in the interest of another – the patient or client. But again, conflicting interests are often at work.

Way wrote in 1962: 'The doctor is never contradicted, and by various means he is shown to be a person of pre-eminent skill and wisdom.' It seems barely possible that this was written only a generation ago. The fact that it was relevant then only shows how quickly certain values can change.

The relationship between nurses and doctors has largely been characterized by social and professional inequality. 'If woman came from Adam's rib, the nurses, I fear, must have come from the physician's rib' (Partridge, 1978). Stereotypes of doctors as men, nurses as women; doctors as middle class, nurses as working class; doctors having a long education, nurses having training; doctors ordering, nurses carrying out orders – such distinctions are disappearing. But in critical situations it is still usually the doctor who has the last word. Is it because he is a man, 'knows better', is more confident, has been trained that way, has (or takes) status?

Questions of inequality are always situations of power. When the ideal of partnership with patients infiltrates also the relationship between nurses and doctors, then something new is happening. Judgements of all concerned are not always easy to resolve.

Nursing autonomy

Autonomy has to do with discretion, control and self-government. Jameton (1984) argues that personal autonomy comes before professional autonomy. He defines an autonomous action as one which is carried out because of goals or values which are attached to it.

Personal and professional autonomy should be egalitarian. Patients, nurses and all health personnel are equals in their own right and should not be dominated by any one group of them. Such autonomy is based on reason, mutual confidence through having listened, identification with the other, and avoidance of coercion to obtain one's own ends (Jameton, 1984). In other words, such autonomy is based on professional ethical standards, and this in turn is based on the relationship with the client or patient.

The *struggle* for autonomy is generally a struggle for power and authority. Although nursing is 'dominated' by doctors, nurses in turn 'dominate' others. The hierarchical structure in nursing serves to maintain this need to dominate, and nurses do it often ferociously to their own kind, as well as to assistants and volunteers and, until recently, housekeeping personnel.

Some nurses do have a large measure of autonomy, notably midwives and community mental health nurses. The case of nurse-practitioners is another example. The suggestion that patients in general practice surgeries should have the choice of seeing either the nurse or the doctor is pointing in the direction of an egalitarian autonomy, or a 'democratization of the health team' (Christman, 1980, in Pearson, 1983).

If we like it or not, nursing and medicine are inextricably linked. Neither of the professions could be completely autonomous. By 'extending' its role (Pearson, 1983) nursing is asserting its autonomy. But it has also been argued that simply being able to take blood and set up intravenous infusions does not make nurses more autonomous. It may simply make them mini-doctors or glorified technicians – and consequently less 'nurses'. Taking on another's job is not the same as acting independently, when that independent action might have been *not* to do that particular job.

One way in which nursing *is* becoming more and more autonomous is through its research. Much research has been carried out in recent years about different aspects of care. This is not always easily converted into practice because of resistance to change. One good example is the use of Eusol. Research has established it as a harmful agent for wound care, yet it is still prescribed by doctors for that use. Nurses aware of such research have a duty to challenge harmful agents such as Eusol, according to the UKCC advisory document *Exercising Accountability*.

Making independent decisions

When nurses become more conscious of their role and ability, and their responsibilities and rights, then making decisions based on these aspects will inevitably be independent if they are viewed from within a framework of control. Some of the cases where nurses have taken decisions not to cooperate with treatments have been well documented, and all the nurses have suffered for their actions.

In 1983 *Nursing Times* reported the case of a nurse who had not called the emergency team after a 78-year-old man had collapsed after an operation, but decided to let the patient 'die peacefully' and for this judgement on her part she was dismissed.

The case of the mental health nurse has already been mentioned (see Chapter 5, page 69). He decided independently that the patient was not fit for ECT and he would not cooperate. A statement by the RCN in relation to this case makes the point that 'it would be naive to imagine that the mantle of accountability can be assumed without accepting that it may demand a high sacrifice' (*Nursing Times*, 1985b).

In a case reported by Lawrence and Crisham (1984) an American nurse was 'suspended from duty for unprofessional conduct'. She was accused of interfering with the doctor–patient relationship when she gave a patient 'information about her condition against the doctor's orders'. A State Supreme Court however 'ruled that her behaviour could not be classified as unprofessional because it violated no specific clause of the Board of Nursing's rules'.

These are only three examples out of many possible ones. No doubt many more happen than are actually reported in the press.

A common link between these examples is that they show up clearly that the nurses involved in each case had a particular relationship with the patient. Each nurse acted out of the understanding she or he had of that relationship. In the first example, the nurse had glimpsed from the relationship with her patient that he had suffered enough. In the second example, the mental health nurse's relationship with his patient led him to concentrate on the physical symptoms and consider these more important than the psychiatric ones. In the last example, the nurse had presumably built up a trusting relationship with her patient in which both were free to talk honestly in a way that the doctor was unable to.

The relationship between nurses and patients is again seen to be the crucial and deciding factor. When decisions about treatments are made on the basis of conservation of life and the scientific results of tests, then clearly something is missing, for the recipient of care is a person, not a machine. An ethic of caring may therefore justly challenge a decision made by a doctor, or make a decision which is based on care more than on cure.

Some of these decisions by nurses to act independently have resulted in changes of practice. A report in *Nursing Times* (1987) cited a document which highlighted the decline in the use of ECT as directly attributable to nurses' actions or resistance.

- Are there practices and treatments which nurses should and could challenge more?

Challenging medical opinion or treatments

Despite assertiveness, less glorification of doctors, and being constantly urged to act in the patient's best interest, it is not easy to challenge a doctor, and win:

> Brian, a 58-year-old man with Down's syndrome, severe deafness, and increasing aortic valve incompetence, lived in a home where he was difficult to manage because of falling and incontinence (both caused by his heart disease). He had a brother and sister-in-law and a 16-year-old nephew who was very fond of him. Two years earlier a cardiac consultant had written in his notes that he should not be operated on as that would be an unfair intrusion into his world. A different consultant thought otherwise, and Brian was admitted for aortic valve replacement. Unfortunately, his family were booked to go on holiday at this time, and after discussion with the surgeon they went, trusting that all would be well. Brian was seen preoperatively by a nurse from the ITU who felt she didn't get through to him. She had talked to the consultant and asked him not to operate. But the operation was carried out, Brian was very sick afterwards, and appeared terrified when he woke up. He was in the ITU for ten days, unable to communicate, without his family, getting increasingly more ill, and finally dying. During this time a hostility built up between the nurses and the consultant which made caring very difficult.

The various aspects of inequality between nurses and doctors are strong arguments why the doctor should win an argument, and the nurse should accept it. But there are equally strong arguments why the opposite should be true. Again and again studies show that nurses are more in touch with patients than doctors, can predict death more accurately because of close contact with patients, and have a healing touch which doctors are not aware of. If, therefore, doctors will not listen to nurses, then nurses have to speak to doctors in a language they can understand. Indeed it has been said that women are better at communicating than men.

Therefore, perhaps nurses should exploit this capacity more often and more deliberately when a patient's health and life is in question.

Downe (1990) asks 'What are you as a midwife supposed to do when the doctor sails into the room where you are looking after your client, says very little, and leaves after writing in the notes 'for ARM at next VE' (artificial rupture of membranes at the next vaginal examination)?' Downe then gives five possible ways of challenging the doctor:

1   Undertake the next VE and claim that the woman is not dilated enough for the policy on routine rupture of membranes to apply.
2   Say to the woman involved: 'I could undertake an ARM, and these are the pros and cons – you don't really want it, do you? and then write in the notes 'X refuses ARM'.
3   Refuse to carry out ARM on the grounds that it is against your professional judgement, based on research evidence.
4   Offer the woman the information for and against ARM in as unbiased a way as possible, and act on her decision, recording the discussion honestly in the notes.
5   Seek to change policy that is not based on research evidence.

These types of responses must be familiar not only to midwives but to nurses of all types. It is possible to take this case and look at it in terms of ethical decision-making.

Step One: Assessment

• What is happening:
  – to the patient?
  – to the midwife?
• What is the role of each person involved:
  – patient?
  – midwife?
  – doctor?
• What obligations has the midwife vis-à-vis:
  – the patient?
  – the doctor?
  – the profession?
• How does she fulfil these?

- Who or what makes the strongest claims on her?
- How does she feel in this situation?
- Has she been in similar situations before? What happened then? What can be learnt from this?
- How does this incident affect her relationship with her patient?
- Which ethical principles are mostly affected:
  - value of life?
  - respect for the person?
  - good and right: beneficence?
  - justice and fairness?
  - truth-telling and honesty?
  - individual freedom: autonomy?
  - non-maleficence?
- How are they affected?
- What does this mean for her present situation?

Step Two:　Planning

- Does the midwife see this situation mainly in terms of:
  - her duty?
  - the outcome of her action?
  - the relationship with her client?
- Which of these is going to guide her decisions?
- What outcomes do any possible actions have?
- Which actions are possible?
- How is any one of the ethical principles furthered or hindered by a particular action?
- What personal values are at stake?
- What could the midwife do not to have such a situation occur again?

It can be seen that of the five possibilities for action outlined above 1 and 2 are both unethical and unprofessional. Possibility 3:

> is confrontational, but at least it expresses the considered view of the professional midwife and recognizes that a nurse or midwife cannot protect herself from charges of professional misconduct by claiming that 'the doctor ordered me to carry out the procedure', if she should reasonably have known that the action was not in the interest of the client (Downe, 1990).

Option 5 is evidently the right thing to do, but cannot be achieved overnight. And it still leaves the nurse with the decision what to *do now*.

Choice 4 is a compromise. But is it right to shift the responsibility onto the patient at a difficult time? It could not be right to leave the patient and run after the doctor to challenge him, therefore a decision will have to be taken. The one which is most responsible under the circumstance is the one which will be the most right, good, just, truthful – and caring.

Step Three: Implementation

• The decision taken will have to be carried out, and recorded.

Step Four: Evaluation

• This will be the test if the decision was the right one. In the light of the evaluation a further step will have to be taken so that the midwife (or nurse) will not be placed in this situation again.

In order to act ethically the midwife does not only have to make the right decision at the moment. She has a professional duty to see that unethical acts are prevented. Thus she should take some action to see that she will not be in this predicament again. But more still: it does not only concern herself. Ethics concerns everybody. What one person does affects others. She should, in seeking change in this area, also seek that all others in similar positions are relieved of difficulties and that a bad practice is eliminated. Thus it can be seen that one person's 'fight' or responsible and accountable act does have wide repercussions.

Whenever nurses (and midwives and health visitors) find themselves in situations which they cannot agree with – which are often caused by prescribed treatments – they need to make this clear. This is essentially, though sometimes indirectly, an act of advocacy.

Nurses have challenged doctors in many areas where they believed treatments were not adequate or appropriate. Nurses in a neonatal unit objected to a research trial which consisted of removing cerebro-spinal fluid from a baby with post-haemor-rhagic hydrocephalus, and returning it to the infant via his artificial milk-feed. Nurses described the practice as 'cannibalistic'

(Lyall, 1989). In another report (*Nursing Times*, 1986) nurses objected to being pressurized by doctors who allowed research trials without the patients' agreement.

Nurses question orders for resuscitation and for not-resuscitation (Stewart and Rai, 1989) and many treatments prescribed for patients who are dying. But to be heard and taken seriously by doctors is still not always easy:

> A lady was brought to the Accident and Emergency department. She had been found unconscious at home by her son, the day after her seventy-sixth birthday. She had swallowed half a bottleful of sleeping tablets, and a bottleful of analgesic tablets. A student nurse was sent to take care of her. A young houseman soon arrived and deliberated with the student whether or not he should treat this lady. The student had argued that she shouldn't be treated, in view of her very poor home circumstances. The doctor then decided that it was his duty to treat the lady, and went ahead, asking the nurse to assist him.

An attempt at consultation between equals was made, but as both nurse and doctor were rather inexperienced, fear of censure, and perhaps personal reputation, won the day.

These stories are not isolated examples of non-cooperation, or asking for advice and then rejecting it, between doctors and nurses. 'As nurses we have little say in the treatment decisions made, but we are the ones that must look after and carry out treatments for these (people), sometimes against our ethical beliefs or simply our natural feelings' (Thornton, 1984).

Nurses cannot only blame doctors – nursing and nurses themselves have much to answer for such situations; relationships involve two parties. Nursing may never be an independent profession, but nursing and medicine should be more truly interdependent. It is not a question of who cares better or cures more.

Nurses have often seen themselves as powerless. But Jameton (1984) points out that nurses often focus their anger, bitterness and frustration with care on the doctors, making them the scapegoats. In this way nurses only reinforce medical dominance and keep doctors at the centre of attention, so reinforcing a stereotyped image of dominator and dominated. The doctor-nurse game is maintained on a merry-go-round. Only when nurses have enough self-knowledge and insight into such games can they be seen for what they are and change for the better. Only when nurses and doctors respect each other as equals with different professional roles is creativity possible.

To show that it can be done, Turner (1989) reported on a geriatric intermediate rehabilitation ward, where nurses challenged the doctors' supremacy and won the day. They depended neither on external funding nor on a selective criteria for patients, but on communication and collaboration.

When a person's professional judgement is questioned by a colleague an element of mistrust is always evident. Personal gain and status are subtle components of most of what we do. Defending a position may have as much to do with experience as with feared or wanted reputation. Motives for acting in certain ways will always have to be questioned because they will always be questioned. The values of communication: attention, intelligence, reasonableness, responsibility and commitment seem particularly called for in such situations.

Ethical issues between nurses and their employers

The employer is the one who hires and fires. To remain in the job, the employee has to dance to his tune.

In a small business or place of work people know each other, and decisions are made by agreement. A large business, however, is mostly anonymous, and this requires not discussion and agreement but obedience (Handy, 1983). Hospitals and health authorities tend to be hierarchical and bureaucratic institutions. The relationship between employee and employer is one of contract and obligation, not one of consensus; it is formal, not friendly. And in a climate of economy, efficiency and effectiveness the individual's needs count less than the corporate needs. Difficulties in the relationship between nurses and their employers focus largely on the needs of the individual versus the needs of the organization. Ideally, the relationship between employer and employee should also be based on the same principles as those between nurse and patient: care, and care based on receptivity, reciprocity and responsivity.

The ethical issues which arise between nurses and employers

arise out of the conflict of what the employer demands and does, and how the nurse responds to this demand.

Standards of care

Most nurses in Britain will by now be acquainted with some form of setting of standards. Qualpacs (Quality Patient Care Scale) and Monitor and Nursing Audit are names which have passed into the language. All these various instruments are quality assurance measures concerned with performance. The Quality Circles are less concerned with a fixed indicator but work more on a personal level where the coordinator and leader play a significant role.

'Standards of care are valid, acceptable definitions of the quality of nursing care' (Sale, 1990). They are often written to solve a problem, but are 'intended to ensure that practice moves forward and does not stagnate'. In order to be viable, standards are 'presented in statements of performance to be achieved within an agreed time, and are acceptable, achievable, observable and measurable'.

In order to set such standards, and to have professional control of them, 'nurses need to be clear about the extent of their authority, responsibility and accountability, which must be matched with the necessary authority to carry out their job effectively'.

Accountability

Accountability can have many definitions. Binnie et al (1984) describe it as 'being personally responsible for the outcome of one's own professional actions'.

According to the UKCC Code a nurse is primarily accountable to the patient and to the public. Binnie et al believe that nurses are also accountable to their colleagues, particularly if they have delegated care to them.

Common sense would dictate that a nurse must also be accountable to her employer, her profession and even herself', says Tingle (1990b) – and rightly so.

Accountability means not only having to answer for an action when something went wrong, but it is a continuous process of monitoring how a nurse performs professionally. The responsibility differs in different situations, but there is a need to be aware that one is constantly responsible, and therefore constantly accountable.

A distinction needs to be made between legal and moral accountability.

The interrelatedness of all humanity – and all nature – means that everyone is responsible for some people, be they family, friends, or patients and clients. This responsibility brings with it an accountability to something bigger than ourselves. Religious people would say that they have to answer to God for the responsibility they have of other people. Others would say that a general sense of morality makes us responsible to humanity at large, or to our own higher self. Legal accountability arises out of the training a person had, and relates to the position held. Thus it is clear that a student nurse has different accountability to a senior manager. But both have a similar degree of moral accountability which relates to the ethical principles, i.e. respect, goodness, justice and honesty.

In order to be legally accountable a nurse needs certain specific things:

- A degree of autonomy.
- A freedom to act or practise in accordance with the training and education.
- To use her or his judgement and to act on it.

Autonomy

Autonomy has been described above (see page 101). Every situation presents its own problems and challenges to be and act autonomously.

Autonomy gives power to a person. The excursions into the extended role of nurses give them more power. But it must be clear what that power is, and what it is being used for. If it means more and better care for a particular patient, then this is right. If it means simply more dominance or distance from caring work with patients and colleagues, it should be questioned.

Freedom to act

Once a person has attained a certain degree of competence, particularly in a profession like nursing, she or he needs to be able to practise that competence.

Carlie was a third-year student nurse in charge of a male surgical ward at night. One of her patients was an elderly man with carcinoma of the prostate who was dying. He had an intravenous infusion and a catheter, and a fluid balance chart was kept. His wife was with him and asked Carlie if she could give her husband sips of tea from her flask. Carlie agreed happily, and all during the long hours of the night the patient received small sips of his favourite drink. When Carlie reported for duty the next night she was called into the night manager's office and asked why the tea had not been recorded on the patient's fluid balance chart.

This is too much like petty punishment to teach a student nurse about accountability. Indeed, Keighley (1986) makes a point which highlights this and the above heading:

Accountability is not a trip wire to catch out the nurse, it is a *dynamic process which guides and determines the role content of nursing* (emphasis added). It makes superfluous a debate about the extended role of the nurse, because it provides the framework for nurses to evolve their role within the principles underlying health care.

- How does accountability become that framework?
- How should accountability be taught?

Use one's judgement

Perhaps this shows accountability most clearly as a need in nursing. More autonomy leads to more assertiveness about one's skills, and this in turn leads to initiating orders, not only following them. The autonomy has to be practised.

Whoever initiates actions has to answer for them. And such actions must then be 'explainable, defendable, and based on knowledge rather than on tradition or myth' (Binnie et al, 1984). Standards of care guide a nurse to what she or he can and should do, and check if they are done. Accountability is that answerability.

Responsibility

The above three headings could be summed up also as responsibility. Whoever has responsibility has accountability. The two are intertwined and not separable (see Table 8.1). Using the word 'responsibility' brings the concept back again to a more caring, even feminine level. Responsibility is never something very clearcut. It can always stretch beyond a boundary, because it is born out of responsivity, reciprocity and receptivity. This is not a danger, because true accountability is that check which quite naturally knows the boundary which is there for both, as it is based on clear, unambiguous and honest communication.

Table 8.1 Defining responsibility and accountability

Responsibility	*Accountability*
Nurses have: • Ethical responsibility • Legal responsibility	Nurses have: • Moral accountability • Legal accountability
There is professional responsibility: • To care • To maintain and improve • To act	Nurses must have authority which comes from training and experience
This is linked to: • Freedom • Goodness • Rightness to act ⟶	arises out of responsibility
Responsibility means to be answerable	
Responsibility goes beyond duty: there is a relational responsibility	Concept has arisen because of: • Awareness • Autonomy • Prescribing care
	Accountability is a continuous process of monitoring: • To client or patient • To profession and public through UKCC • To colleagues (person above us) • To self

Accountability in action

Accountability to the employer is perhaps the most difficult to sustain strictly. With ever tighter budgets managers are squeezed on every side. In the way of things, everyone tends to look after his/her own interests and squeezes the one below. The following is a story of being squeezed.

Eve was a 50-year-old staff nurse who had done two or three nights a week on a male medical ward for the last twenty years or so. It was a provincial hospital, and she had never changed wards, although at night she often went to other wards to cover for nurses on their meal breaks. About a year previously all staff had received a letter to say that they were in future not appointed to a ward but to the hospital so that they could be deployed wherever the need was greatest. Eve had read the letter but dismissed it thinking this would not apply to her in her position.

It was the night of Boxing Day, and Eve's ward promised to be very quiet with few patients, and those they had were sleeping well after the festivities.

She had just started to settle one particularly heavy patient when she was called to the telephone and asked to go to the children's ward where the regular nurse had not come in after a slight accident on her way in. Eve protested; not her surely, she had not handled a sick child since her training days. Even at night she never went to the children's ward as they always covered for each other separately there. The senior nurse insisted, as there was no other qualified nurse available and Eve's ward was quiet.

Eve went reluctantly, leaving a nursing assistant, and a second-year student nurse who was sent to replace her. She glanced at each child's records as she had a quick walking report from the student nurse on the ward. There were twelve children, mostly very sick, some with a parent beside them. They welcomed her as they were alarmed at the prospect of not having a qualified nurse at night.

Eve felt less reassured. After an hour she had an admission of a child who had had a fit. When she had time later she visited a child who had been very quiet and nobody had taken too much notice of because of the extra work. This child now had vomit all around him and Eve picked him up quickly and ran with him in her arms to the telephone to call the emergency team. Their arrival caused a commotion and one of the babies dislodged a drip, causing another emergency. When morning finally came, one of the older children was missing. Trying to pull herself together in a moment during the various dramas, Eve had gone to the sluice and opened the door to the fire escape for some fresh air. She forgot to close it, and the child, half asleep, had wandered unobserved during the various emergencies, and was discovered by the porter collecting rubbish bags, asleep on the fire escape.

Similar stories must be more and more common where nurses are asked to take over duties for which they are not trained or prepared.

Clause 4 of the UKCC Code is clear that 'each registered nurse, midwife and health visitor is accountable for his or her practice, and, in the exercise of professional accountability shall . . . acknowledge any limitations of competence and refuse in such cases to accept delegated functions'. Eve should have referred to this clause and not accepted to go to the children's ward as she clearly was not competent to work there. But the pressure for her to go was great. Her possibilities were:

1 To refuse to go on the spot.
2 To go but decline any responsibility.
3 After the event to make her objection known.

Option 1 would have been the most honest. Option 2 was not really possible, as once engaged on the job, she was responsible. Option 3 should be done anyway.

Accountability is not only owning up to mistakes, but it is also preventing them. In this sense accountability can be seen to be both deontological (doing the dutiful thing rightly) and teleological (forestalling any harmful consequences).

If Eve had refused to go to the children's ward this would have left the night manager in a difficult situation. She might simply have called on another nurse to do the same, and put her or him into the same position. This is essentially dishonest because while it leaves her untouched, others are put into situations of compromise.

This situation is different only in context to the one described above of the midwife. Each example shows that a nurse is constantly accountable to the patient, the profession, the public, her colleagues and herself.

The UKCC advisory document *Exercising Accountability* (1989) elaborates on several of the clauses in the UKCC Code which concern a nurse's accountability.

Conflict with managers

Some ethical difficulties between nurses and employers are less clearcut than the above example. In the present climate of value-for-money and applying the language of business to health care, many managers of small and large units are administrators and managers with no experience of hospitals, health care or nursing. It is quite possible that a nurse's manager is not another nurse. That manager too is concerned to fulfil his or her expected standards, and these may differ from the nurse's.

Saving money through ward closures, cutting services and 'rationalizing' duty rotas is not always what a nurse sees as obvious means to fulfil that aim. Many such practices mean more work for nurses who are already understaffed. It may be that the nurses available are enough in numbers on a piece of paper, but they have neither the skills nor the experience for that particular work. It is not always easy to make this clear to a manager. Many nurses feel indignant about being told how to run a ward or unit by someone without any similar experience.

Any type of coercion inevitably undermines and limits a person's autonomy, freedom and judgement. Coercion achieves only an unwilling compliance, and this is playing with power. This is possible at many levels and is a subtle form of manipulation.

- What are the motives when someone uses coercion rather than communication?
- Could and should these motives be challenged?

1991 saw the postponed implementation of the White Paper *Working for People*. As with any new way of working this will demand a great deal of ingenuity and flexibility. It can only be hoped that it will lead to cooperation more than confrontation. The hastily introduced GP contract caused a great deal of concern for GPs, practice nurses and their patients and yet another change will not be easy unless accompanied by goodwill.

The notions of responsibility and accountability are good and helpful in the abstract. However, when things go wrong, communication is not open and relationships are not fostered, then they become weapons with which to defend positions. They may be used legitimately for this, but it should not be forgotten that they stem from a wider ethic of caring which is creative, responsive and tending towards another who is addressed as Thou.

Objection to treatments and policies

When nurses object to certain treatments they don't only come into conflict with the prescribing doctor, but also with their employer. At present a nurse can only legally object to taking part in abortion. The 'conscience clause' in the Abortion Act (1967) is there for that purpose. Further than that, a nurse is professionally duty-bound to give treatments as ordered to a patient. (An abortion is not strictly speaking a 'treatment'.)

An act of conscientious objection or civil disobedience is non-cooperation with the law. The law permits abortion, but a nurse may object to it on moral or religious grounds; in other words, she or he does not have to cooperate with the law.

Objecting to abortion may be compared with objecting to war or refusing to pay taxes. Abortions, like wars, will still go on, and one person's objection may be another person's unwilling partaking, because *someone* has to do it. By objecting to abortion the issue will not go away. In this sense, objecting to a law may be seen simply as a selfish act.

Some nurses will have thought deeply about the subject and would *prefer* not to take part in abortions, or other morally ambiguous procedures, but feel that to remain involved and take part may be more realistic.

In recent years nurses have objected to ECT as a 'treatment'. They have at times objected to nursing patients with AIDS. This is where it is important to be clear about the difference between objection to a treatment, conscientious objection and making moral judgements about a person's lifestyle. Indeed, in this latter case nurses were warned that if they refused to treat patients with AIDS they were liable to be removed from the register.

Many nurses feel that so-called treatments given to very ill or dying patients are objectionable. But they do not have the *right* to refuse to carry them out. They can, and should, question the prescriptions if they feel they cannot comply with them. There may also be situations where health professionals collude with patients' relatives for interventions which the patient might not want, such as an abortion for an under-age girl or the imposition of ECT on a reluctant patient (Crabbe, 1988).

Nurses who find themselves in such situations face a real dilemma. Can they truly be the patient's advocate? Do they know that the patient has enough information to make an independent decision?

Nurses often feel isolated in such cases. They may hold values and views which others might not share, and which might be considered old-fashioned or selfish. They may fear that they will be labelled as troublemakers.

Managers faced with a nurse who cannot agree with certain treatments can easily coerce a nurse into complying, citing inexperience. This 'hierarchical terror' does not help, however. Too many nurses have left the job disillusioned, guilty, anxious and unheard.

- What responsibilities does the profession as a whole have to challenge uncaring attitudes in managers?

So often, nurses have to make ethical decisions on the spot, and do not have the privilege of consulting codes and books before acting. It may, therefore, be an opportunity to take the problem of objecting to a prescribed treatment and look at it here in terms of ethical decision-making.

Step One: Assessment

- What is happening?
- What is the actual treatment?
- Why is it questionable?
- Who are the people involved?
- What is the involvement of each?

- What relationships do they have to each other?
- What is good about the situation?
- What is bad about the situation?
- Which particular ethical principle is involved?
  - value of life
  - goodness or rightness/beneficence
  - justice
  - truth-telling
  - individual freedom/autonomy
  - respect of the person
  - non-maleficence
- What feelings are particularly strong or evident?
- Has everybody been able to say freely everything he/she needed to say?

Step Two: Planning

- What would happen if the treatment continued/were carried out?
- What would happen if the treatment did not continue/were not carried out?
- Is it a question of:
  - duty (whose?)
  - consequences?
  - maintaining or fostering relationships?
- Which one of these do the various people involved feel most strongly appertains to them?
- What does a duty involve in this instance?
- What consequences are possible/foreseeable?
- Do any of the actions or consequences have some meaning for any person involved, i.e. are they linked to some memory or goal?
- Have all the aspects of:
  - compassion
  - competence
  - confidence
  - conscience
  - commitment
  been understood and taken into consideration?
- What actions are possible?

- What actions are likely to be most effective:
  - how?
  - why?
  - when?
  - where?
- What else needs to be decided, and by whom?
- Who will take what action, and when, where and how?

Step Three: Implementation

The action is carried out.

Step Four: Evaluation

- Have the predictions come true?
- If not, why not?
- What might have been done better?
- Is the outcome satisfactory?
- If not, why not?
- What else has happened which was not foreseen?
- How does this fit into the scheme of things?
- What are the various relationships now?

These are inevitably only some questions which might be asked, and they do not yet constitute the actual plan of action. Such a plan may contain some of the following:

- Talking more with the patient.
- Talking with the relatives.
- Talking with colleagues.
- Talking with the doctor.
- Finding out what happened in similar situations before.
- Planning a case conference.
- Meeting with senior nurses.
- Writing a letter to management.
- Contacting the UKCC for advice.
- Setting up a committee for monitoring the situation.
- Setting up a support group.

When a nurse is in a situation of conflict, she or he needs support and help, not censure. If this support comes from senior management this is ideal. The fact is that it will more likely come from peers and even from outside her immediate colleague circle. But support should be there, otherwise a nurse may not be able to cope with a situation. Employers have a duty to support their staff; and staff are responsible to the employer to carry out care as well as possible. When these are both happening, then all concerned will be satisfied.

Stover and Nightingale (1985) cite many examples of torture and psychiatric abuse of people where nurses were involved, sometimes willingly, sometimes against their will. Codes and declarations ask nurses not only not to participate, but to expose such practice. But this is far from easy. Gross abuse is more easily recognized, but more subtle forms of misconduct may also infringe human rights and eventually lead to a blurring of vision of what is and what is not legitimate. The 'discovery' in 1989 of the conditions on Leros, the Greek island where psychiatric patients were kept in sub-human conditions (Carlisle, 1989), is only one example of what is still possible today.

Unwarranted treatment, treatments labelled 'research', too much or too little pain control and abusive treatments (such as disciplining patients with cold showers) (Jameton, 1984) must be questionable at least and ask of nurses, in the name of humanity, to object to them.

Because nurses recognized abuses of human rights in their more subtle forms and objected to them out of their own understanding of human rights, human needs and human relationships, changes have taken place. The pioneers in these fields – as with any pioneers – have a hard, uphill struggle because they go against or beyond the known and the recognized. But caring is not only restoring something ill to good health, it is wider and more far-reaching, and caring includes the prevention of ill-health, therefore boundaries have to be stretched outwards. Change *can* be brought about when the need is recognized, and nurses are prepared to fight and know how to make it happen.

In wanting greater autonomy as professionals, in wanting to fulfil the roles of advocates and change agents, nurses will need to consider also those areas of conscientious objection to abuse of too much or too little legitimate care. By going beyond boundaries which are sometimes quite arbitrarily imposed or exist for the comfort of officialdom only, nurses are truly caring, human persons.

Ethical issues between nurses and nurses

Most of the ethical issues which arise between nurses are to do with incidences of assault, abuse or theft. Should a nurse tell on another nurse? What are her or his obligations?

> Mary was a senior enrolled nurse who had been working on a particular geriatric ward for many years. The patient was a woman with Parkinson's disease, and occasionally suffered from sharp edges to her tongue. Mary had just finished bathing this lady when she got rather a mouthful from her. Indignant, Mary returned the insult by smacking the patient's bottom. She realized at once what she had done and went and told Omar, the charge nurse, asking him not to reveal this to anyone else. Omar consented to this. But unbeknown to both, Linda, a young staff nurse, had witnessed the act and had gone straight to the nursing office to report the incident. Mary was immediately suspended from duty and shortly afterwards dismissed.

Most nurses would say that they are first and foremost loyal to patients. But this can sometimes backfire.

This story shows not only various types of loyalties, but also various types of actions and responsibilities, obligations and contraventions.

Another story highlights another aspect of the same problem:

> Frances had been newly appointed to the post of ward sister. She noticed that one of her staff nurses often had a peculiar smell about her after the morning break. One day she received a telephone call from the person who had held the post before her, and who was now a nurse manager in a different health authority; she said that the strange smell was due to a kind of medication this staff nurse rubbed into her painful knees. She wanted to be sure that the new sister was aware of this staff nurse's personal difficulties. Some time later, however, the staff nurse was admitted to hospital with a liver complaint due to alcoholism.

There have been many reports over the years of nurses accusing other nurses of abuse and even brutality (e.g. *Nursing Times*, 1989;

Heywood Jones, 1989). In most of these reports there are clear indications that nurses were 'too terrified' to report the incident because they had been threatened by the person concerned, or that a senior nurse or manager to whom it was reported took no notice and even seemed to condone the treatment.

Students in particular are very vulnerable to threats if they make a complaint. They have to consider their reports, their education and indeed their careers. They find it often particularly difficult to challenge those in charge of them.

> Dick was a charge nurse on a psychiatric ward where primary nursing was used successfully. Due to reorganization there was no senior nurse for his unit in post. Dick had formed a very strong and supportive relationship with one of his patients, Anne. They spent much time together and Anne improved considerably. Because of aspects of confidentiality, Dick could not easily talk about Anne at the reports, and other staff began to resent the fact that Dick and Anne spent so much time together, feeling that other patients (and they themselves) were thereby neglected. Because there was no senior nurse, his colleagues went to higher authority to voice concern. This was noted, but no action taken.

> One day when they were short staffed, and Dick and Anne were together in his office, a drug error was made on the ward. This proved to be the straw which broke the camel's back, and Dick was formally warned that he might be dismissed for unprofessional behaviour. Anne was discharged within a few days, and shortly after this she and Dick announced their engagement. The warning of dismissal was automatically dropped.

Marriage may be an answer to difficult situations, but it must be a very unusual one! In an interesting article McCarthy (1986) highlights many of the issues behind the acts of maltreatment of patients by nurses and the feelings involved. He points out that nurses, who are meant to be 'nice' people who protect their patients, can have very ambivalent feelings when witnessing an attack. 'Revulsion, excitement, anger, fascination, shock, sorrow and impotence' are some of the feelings listed. It is not surprising that nurses then feel guilty, rationalize what happened, and with a lack of confidence – because of their reactions – feel unable to take the issue further.

But just as regularly as nurses report feeling terrified about blowing the whistle on colleagues, the UKCC Professional Conduct Committee tells nurses that 'the overriding principle at stake in misconduct is the nurse's duty towards the patient' (Anonymous, 1989). The UKCC Code, Clause 1 ('Act always in such a way as to promote and safeguard the wellbeing and interests of patients/clients') is cited as the guideline.

The process for making the decision about whether an incident should be reported or not is similar to that for objecting to treatments (see page 117).

Loyalty to colleagues is a noble thing. But sometimes a misguided loyalty is only a loyalty to one's own inadequacy.

Abuse, assault, or any kind of malpractice is never excusable. But what is not excusable either is that the accused is not given a hearing. No one commits such acts without some reason which may be deeply hidden. While nurses may be in trouble with their employers and the profession, they *must* also be given help and support by the employer and the profession to get back into acceptable ways. The relationship between a nurse and 'the profession' is a loose one, but some*one* in that profession must be available to form a helping, caring and creative relationship with the member of the profession who has thus become its casualty.

Ethical issues between nurses and the profession

The saying 'once a nurse, always a nurse' is losing its legitimacy. The spirit of it may still hold true, but not the letter of it. The introduction of periodic registration and updating by PREPP (Post-Registration Education and Practice Project) means that nurses have accepted that to remain practising they have to continue learning and improving their skills.

But skills training is not enough. To practise any job or profession means to give the best service within given frameworks or limits. To step outside these limits may be harmful to the client and the professional.

Some of the issues which cause difficulties between nurses and the profession are to do with the understanding of what the 'profession' means and does. Some of it has to do with the image

presented by professionals, and some of it has to do with politics
with a small p and a large P.

Political action

Should nurses be involved in politics? Perhaps the question is
rather, can they afford not to be?

Every nurse in the NHS is employed because some government
official has sanctioned that particular post. These officials are the
very ones who hold the purse strings of some health authority.
From there come directives regarding economy, efficiency and
effectiveness. An official can give directives, but it is the nurse
who, at the end of the chain of command, carries them out. Seen
in this way, nurses are political pawns, their actions are political
and their jobs are political.

Many nurses – and other health care workers – feel that to
defend their rights they need to belong to a union or professional
body. These organizations exist to speak on behalf of nurses and
defend their interests, such as conditions of work, pay, etc. This
leaves the actual workers free to get on with their own jobs.

But many nurses find that this is not enough for them. There
are some notable nurses in both Houses of Parliament, and some
professional organizations of all kinds have made themselves be
talked about. However, the exclusion of the chief nursing officer
from the NHS Policy Board in 1989 was regarded as a grave
mistake by nurses. Despite vigorous protests at the time, the then
Secretary of State for Health did not change his mind. It took a
new Secretary of State in 1990 to reverse that decision, and he
can only be applauded.

In order not to keep but to advance the autonomy nurses have
they need to be at the forefront of every policy. They need not
only to be there when policies are being made, but they need to
put them forward. They need to be instrumental in change. That
is inevitably costly in terms of time and energy.

● How costly is it *not* to act?

Many times policies have to be challenged. The politics of the
'free market' means that occasionally one person's or organization's ends become another's means, and that is not acceptable.
Some examples of this were a trial proposed by the Medical

Research Council in 1986 for elderly men suffering from prostate cancer to undergo castration. Once this had become known, nurses were very quick to condemn the practice and the trial was dropped. Similarly, when the government had approved secret blood tests for HIV from certain people in at-risk groups, nurses declared that they would not cooperate, and the policy was consequently changed. The UKCC issued guidelines to nurses which should be followed whenever a query arises.

On the other hand, more and more nurses are training in one or more of the complementary therapies such as reflexology, aromatherapy, therapeutic touch, etc. and incorporating this in their care (Rankin-Box, 1988). These therapies are usually of the 'low tech–high touch' type and suit the expanding aspect of nursing very well. As complementary therapies take a totally different approach to health and illness from allopathic medicine, nurses who practise these therapies could at present find themselves in difficulty with the professional bodies. Or they could seek that these therapies be regarded as valid and be encouraged in view of the fact that they are holistic in character and would therefore suit an ethic of caring particularly well.

The issues just discussed are not necessarily directly questions of right or wrong or good or bad, and they do not touch so many nurses as some others. Nevertheless, they all have to do with rights in the sense of the importance of equality and not taking advantage of privileged positions. When this *does* happen, the challenge has to be that much harder and wider because it is often based on elitism, whereas nursing is based on care and partnership.

Strikes

One area where nurses do run into difficulties with their profession is on the question of strikes.

The contract between employer and employee implies that there are two sides to a bargain. There is a duty and a right on both sides. Strikes can take place when one side of the bargain is not kept. In most instances, this means that nurses feel they are not adequately remunerated for the service they give.

When nurses strike for more money they put themselves first. Although many people feel that nurses should be paid more, this may not be as effective as when they strike to protest over inadequate provisions for patients. Pulling at the heartstrings of people has more punch than pulling at the purse strings of governments.

Nurses do have rights: the right to a just wage, the right to work in adequate facilities, and the right to defence against being unjustly exploited. But nurses also have a moral duty to recognize the rights of patients (Thompson, Melia and Boyd, 1983) including the right to adequate treatment and to adequate facilities. An American nurse wrote after five weeks on strike, 'It is for these people (her patients and former patients) who have trusted me to provide them with the best possible care that I am striking. I want to feel good about myself as a professional nurse, and the only way I can do that is to be sure the conditions under which I work are good enough for my patients' (Yeager, 1977).

Members of the RCN have pledged themselves not to take strike action. Other health service unions, such as NUPE (National Union of Public Employees) and COHSE (Confederation of Health Service Employees) have not taken the same line, and permit strike action.

It can be argued that 'striking or not striking' is really a question about the status of nurses. If nurses want to be professionals, then they have to act and look like professionals, and share with the clients their knowledge and be committed to their care. These values cannot easily be compatible with strike action.

Going on strike has usually been a worker's last weapon against an employer. But withholding labour in a shop is morally different from withholding care from sick people. Nevertheless, if one or more nurses do have a genuine grievance against a local or district health authority they need to have that last possibility open to them. Nurses who genuinely feel – and have documents to prove – that their management is incompetent or neglectful cannot appeal to them for help. They need to go further. There have to be ways open for this.

This is one area where all sides might use the UKCC Code for their defence, citing Clauses 1, 2, 10 and 11 in particular. Everyone – nurse, health authority, UKCC – is concerned for the wellbeing of patients.

- Whose ends are whose aims?
- How can it be clarified?

In recent times nurses in Britain have not gone on long strikes. They have been more likely to hold mass meetings during meal breaks and attract as much attention as they can in that way. In voicing their grievances they are as concerned about breaching the Code as they are of losing their jobs. This latter could be seen as intimidation and this is not acceptable either. As usual, finding a creative solution is more acceptable than confrontation.

Professionalism

It may be useful to end this chapter with a short analysis of professionalism. This is the substance which binds all these various topics together.

A profession is distinguished by three factors: it teaches its students itself in a body of specific knowledge that must be higher than necessary for ordinary survival; and it regulates its own control over admission to, and dismissal from, the profession. But 'the most distinguishing feature of a profession is the existence of a set of ethical principles regulating the conduct of the professional towards the patient or client' (Havard, 1985). These ethical principles concern particularly the areas of personal and professional interest, and enjoin on the professional never to prefer his own interests above those of his client or patient. The dismissal from the profession of any particular person happens mostly because he has violated this principle, in other words he has not behaved 'professionally'.

The distinction between a doctor (a member of a profession) and a plumber (a member of a trade) is that the professional has an extra injunction: he 'shares with his client what he has to give' (Sieghart, 1985) whereas the tradesman gives a service.

Sometimes a distinction is made between 'profession' and 'professional'. Nursing is not a profession, but nurses see themselves as *professionals* in that they maintain proper standards, are businesslike and prefer the interest of their clients to their own.

Many of the writers on professionalism (Eriksson, 1976; Kratz, 1984; Oakley, 1984; Carr, 1985 and others) point to the aspect of communication between patient and nurse as the major issue on which nursing and professionalism depend. The 'extra dimension' of a profession is to share with the client what it has, and to prefer the client's interests to its own.

Altruism is the hallmark of a profession, and is that which gives it its mystique. However, when the inevitable egoism underneath it becomes evident, not much can save it. 'Angels' can turn into 'fallen angels' frightfully quickly when they demand more money and strike for it.

Cox (1979) suggests that nurses do not act decisively enough because they do not communicate well enough. In the decade or so since she wrote, much has changed: nurses are more vocal as a group; they are taking ideas such as autonomy, advocacy and accountability seriously; books by nurses for nurses have proliferated. All this is splendid. What matters, ultimately, though is that nurses still talk *with* patients, and even more importantly, listen to them. When that happens, then nurses *are* truly advocates, autonomous and accountable. These need to go together with nursing research, so that head and heart will always complement each other.

Most of the topics covered in this chapter relate to professionalism in one way or another. At a conference in Australia in 1988 Baroness McFarlane said that 'professional purity and faithfulness has been replaced by disorder and disarray' in the UK. She blamed management for stifling accountability. She then went on to list her maxims for liberation and a way out of the disarray:

- Breaking current patterns of care and encompassing new ideas.
- Acknowledging the complexity and untidiness of nursing.
- A need for multidisciplinary discussion and research.
- Exposing staff and students to moral conflict to learn ethical decision-making skills.
- Distinguishing between enduring values in nursing and what is an overlay of tradition.
- Fostering creativity and autonomy (*Nursing Times*, 1988).

This sounds remarkably similar to many of the things said in this book! Real professionalism is indeed a healthy balance of both masculine and feminine aspects of care, and when all is said and done, what counts is the relationship between a nurse and the patient, or as Carr (1985) puts it:

> A genuine professional nurse is a person who . . . responds to an individual sick person rather than 'a patient' by availability and attendance (listening as well as talking) and by

communication which includes interest, acceptance of the
person as he (or she) is rather than as she (or he) might like
him (or her) to be, empathy and, where appropriate, touch.

9

Ethical dilemmas

Problems, dilemmas and an ethic of caring

The difference between a problem and a dilemma is that a problem can be solved, but a dilemma cannot be solved: there is only a choice between two equally difficult, or bad, alternatives. This is the case with many of life's situations. There is often no real choice – or rather if there is a choice, the consequences are not bearable; so there is no choice. Most of these situations centre round the beginning or end of life. It is significant that this rarely concerns our own life, but the lives of people around us, and who we are responsible for and responsive to.

Some of the dilemmas around the beginning and end of life are looked at here. It is never possible to cover all aspects, and this is not intended. Those which do not figure are not, therefore, any less important.

An ethic of caring must surely be most appropriate at times and places where either ethics or caring are most vulnerable. The importance of the relationship between care-giver and care-receiver has been stressed strongly throughout this book. It seems then that in situations of real human dilemmas, the real human dimension of relationship should be considered as a vital aspect of the debate. This is not easy, because it is intangible, not measurable and has no basis in law. But against this it can be said that the person who is the significant protagonist is, in the end, always left with a *feeling*. The fact is an act done – an abortion, a ventilator unplugged – and that can be rationalized.

What goes on, sometimes for years, is the irrational: the feeling of guilt, loss and perhaps incompleteness. The relationships that the main person has, therefore, are of crucial importance for looking at these intangible and 'irrational' feelings. Feelings are not wrong; they simply *are*, and because of that they are important. In caring, they matter equally with the tangible and rational aspects.

Considering the relationship aspect in ethical dilemmas is making a case for the feminine side of caring. The masculine side – the legal, logical side – is as important, but cannot have sole priority.

At the beginning of life

Philosophers and theologians through the ages have argued about when life begins. Much of that may have been speculation and more a matter of interest than necessity until recently. With the advent of modern science, this has become a much more debated and debatable topic. The difficulty is that philosophy and theology are often at odds with biology.

The Christian churches have maintained that life begins at conception. The Roman Catholic church has always been concerned with the doctrine of 'ensoulment', or when the new life receives the soul from God. This 'cannot be a process or a gradual development, since the human soul has no material component parts, being a simple spiritual substance, which is present either fully or not at all' (Mahoney, 1984). It is difficult to say that the soul 'enters' the life formed at conception because so many (some sources believe 30 per cent and more) conceptions are aborted before implantation.

The question 'when does life begin?' was deliberately not asked in the *Warnock Report* (Report of the Committee of Enquiry into Human Fertilization and Embryology, 1984), but the legislation based on that report had to make a decision. It is arbitrary to say that life begins at such-and-such a moment, because biological life is a continuum. The debate depends very much on the terms used for describing what is meant by certain ideas.

Ford (1988), a Roman Catholic theologian, has suggested a clear 'line' after much research of various disciplines. He declares that life begins at around fourteen or fifteen days after fertilization is completed, this being the stage when the primitive streak forms.

This – fourteen days – is now also the limit in Britain up until which embryo research is permissible (see page 153). For Ford 'fertilization is not the beginning of the development *of* the human individual but represents the beginning of development *into* a human individual' (IME Bulletin, 1989a). The Roman Catholic church has sometimes argued that an embryo is not a potential human being, but a human being with potential. Mahoney (1984) feels that it would be more true to say that 'the ensouled fetus has promise'. Thus these two theologians are saying similar things.

It is quite significant though, that women often seem to have a completely different approach to when life begins. A number of women who had all been pregnant were asked when they considered that life had begun for their child. The spontaneous answer from all of them was when the child first moved or 'quickened' (around the sixteenth or eighteenth week of pregnancy). This, for the women concerned, was when life really began, i.e. when they could form a relationship with the growing child. Before then, 'life' was abstract; from then on it was *real*.

The ethical dilemmas people are faced with revolve then around their understanding of life and what this entails.

Abortion

Abortion must be the oldest regularly performed operation – often with drastic results. It became known only after the fall of Ceauçescu in Romania, that the country's strict anti-abortion and public health laws meant that among women the main reasons for hospitalization were attempted abortion or the late gynaecological consequences of unsafe abortion.

Abortion is not an issue which makes the headlines any more in Britain. The Abortion Act (1967) allows termination of pregnancy up to the twenty-eighth week of gestation. After lengthy debates in Parliament this was reduced in 1990 to twenty-four weeks. There were strong lobbies to reduce this even further because with advancing technology babies born alive at around those dates stand a fair chance of survival. Nowadays, fewer abortions take place in NHS hospitals and many more in private clinics. Because of this possibility, many women from abroad come to Britain to have their pregnancies terminated here. Despite freely available birth control, abortions have increased steadily since the introduction of the Act.

The ethos of the Abortion Act (1967) is to save life and prevent suffering. The conditions set out for this in the Act are so worded that wide interpretation is possible.

Both pro-abortion and anti-abortion groups tend to be categorical in their methods and defend their principles to the exclusion of any compromise.

Anti-abortion groups like 'Life' maintain in their statements that all abortion is wrong and they base this on the unquestioned principle of the sanctity of life. This argument makes it difficult to reason for the saving of the mother's life, or to consider the kind of life either mother or baby will have. Sanctity, or sacredness of life are religious terms. But they are also implicit in the Hippocratic tradition. In the controversy about abortion they are often used to imply an *absolute* prohibition on the taking of life, or that life should be *absolutely* protected. Ethical principles exist to assert human life and to protect it; they are never absolutes. Society, through its laws, works out the conventions and rules which make these principles operable in practice.

Pro-abortion groups are often feminist in outlook and they base their assumptions on the principle of individual freedom, and on general human rights, in particular the right of the woman over her own body. They maintain this right so absolutely that possibly they argue it to the point of disregarding a growing fetus altogether.

Nurses rightly feel that abortion is an issue of ethical debate for them. They are concerned with preserving and enhancing human life, not destroying it. The 'conscience clause' (see Chapter 8) means that a nurse can opt out of taking part in the actual abortion, but a nurse working in a gynaecological ward is still duty-bound to care for a woman before and after the operation.

Nurses in gynaecological wards have little contact with patients who have abortions; the operation is quick and the patients rarely need to stay longer than a day. This does not mean that it is value-free work for nurses. Abortion is possible 'on demand' and many women are young – even very young – and some appear regularly on the ward. This makes one question the personal and social background of the patients, and it is easy to judge and label them. A relationship is at best fleeting, and that is often unsatisfactory for nurses.

To have an abortion is always a decision which is made under duress. An unwanted pregnancy is an enormous emotional burden. For many women the proposition presents itself without them having thought about the moral implications beforehand. Having to make a decision quickly does not allow them time to think and talk enough. The main factor is the operation itself. It is therefore not surprising that many women suffer emotionally for many years after an abortion, often silently, because they are ashamed or feel guilty, or simply because no one else knows about it and they dare not talk about it because of that.

At the bedside of women undergoing abortion the nurse needs, therefore, to demonstrate a special kind of insight into the pressures which may have led to the decision. Many women are well enough aware of their shortcomings or mistakes, and caring for them ethically means caring for them creatively. This may sound paradoxical in the circumstances; it may also be the beginning of a good recovery process.

It may not be at the bedside that nurses help a person to understand the implications of abortion. But many nurses in family planning clinics, as tutors, and as colleagues are called upon to help someone decide whether to have an abortion or not, or have to decide this for themselves. Under pressure the thoughts are never too clear, the issues and feelings often too entangled to make a decision which is then reversed the next day.

It may be useful to look at abortion in the light of the decision-making process (see Chapter 7) and assume that this is done helping someone to decide whether or not to have an abortion.

Step One: Assessment

- What is happening?
- What has happened?
- Who is involved? How?
- What are the main needs of each person?
- State the problem in terms of each ethical principle:
  - of the value of life/respect for the person
  - of being good and doing right
  - of justice
  - of truth
  - of freedom with regard to (a) the mother and (b) the fetus.
- Which of these principles is particularly important here? Why?

- Has the person had to make a very important decision before? What was it? How had she handled it then? What can be learnt from that for now?
- Does the person feel she has a relationship with the fetus? Does this influence her? How?
- What are the feelings experienced by:
  - the mother
  - the fetus (if possible)
  - the father
  - the helper
  - the immediate circle of family and friends?
- How do these feelings influence what is happening?
- How do the feelings help/hinder?
- How may the main persons involved feel in six months, one year, five years?
- What moral and religious values are important?
- Who will benefit most, and how?
- Who will be hurt, and how?
- Have all the aspects been examined, or what has been left unsaid so far?

Step Two: Planning

At this stage, when everything has been laid out as facts, the question is simply to have an abortion or not.

- Or are there other options?

Review the various criteria:

- Is it a question of duty, i.e. what ought I to do as a citizen (mother, daughter, nurse, etc.)? What obligations do I have, and to whom?
- Is it a question of what the consequences will be, i.e. can I live with my decision? If not, why not?
- Is it a question of responding most creatively and humanly to this situation? What am I gaining from this? How can I use it to help others?
- What can be done now to lessen the emotional impact later?
- Could someone else's experience help?
- If an abortion is the decision, where, when, how is it to be? What arrangements need to be made?

- If the decision is not to have an abortion, what arrangements need to be made?
- Who needs to know of the decision?
- What other aspects, so far not mentioned, could be important?

Step Three: Implementation

If Step Two is well done, then a decision will be firm, and the person will feel good about it. Step Three is then only the logical consequence.

Step Four: Evaluation

In this case, the evaluation will start immediately after the decision is made.

The abortion itself should present no problems, but the feelings surrounding it will be what a person is left with.

Assuming that the operation went well:

- What feeling is the person experiencing?
- Is this a normal reaction?
- Is she feeling as she thought she would? If not, what has changed?
- Is the support sufficient?
- Has it helped to work through the decision-making in this way?

There may be different aspects which are not outlined here which are important, or those mentioned here may not be relevant. What matters in any situation is that as far as possible, it is caring, helpful, responsible and creative. This means that the person can live with the decision and will not suffer through coercion or lack of interest.

It is never possible to be categorical about any personal matter. Abortion is personal, and it is also legal. But that doesn't yet make it right for a particular person. Perhaps the only categorical thing that can be said here is that as professionals we should not take part in illegal abortions (Horan and Jackson, 1984).

Malformed and handicapped babies

Much of the research in embryology has brought about dramatic results and genetic malformation of a fetus can be diagnosed early. When parents are informed of such a possibility they are given the choice of an abortion. Equally, it is possible that hereditary diseases transmitted through, or affecting, one sex only can be detected at a very early stage of an in-vitro fertilization and only the non-affected pre-embryos can be transferred to the mother for gestation. These practices are laudable, but like all such processes at the limits of life, have an ethical dimension to them.

- Is there not a danger of the creation of a 'super-race', with the Nazi experiments not too far away?
- Is it right to invest vast sums of money in practices which at best benefit only very few people?

Such questions may never have a satisfactory answer to them. Economy, efficiency and effectiveness – if seen only in terms of money – will always be in opposition to compassion, competence, confidence, conscience and commitment. In the end it is not a figure at the bottom of a balance sheet which counts, but how that particular person was treated. And despite every advanced treatment and diagnostic tool available, babies are still born malformed and ill with diseases, needing care and love. Many such babies would not have survived long in the past, but the treatments available now also mean that whether and how to treat them has become not only a question of equipment and human and monetary resources, but ethics: should it be done?

- Have handicapped babies a right to life?

In a closely-argued article Kuhse and Singer (1985) say that handicapped babies do not have *more* of a right to life than healthy babies. They follow reasoning which suggests that 'to have a right to something, one must have an interest in it, and to have an interest in continuing to exist, one must be a "continuing self", that is, a being which has at some time had the concept of itself existing over time'. Since severely handicapped newborns cannot claim that right, their right to life cannot be based on potential either.

Is it ever acceptable to treat severely handicapped babies simply to have them live a little longer? Surely not. But where to draw the line and when to call a halt is extremely difficult. Kuhse and Singer conclude that 'there is no fundamental moral reason against thinking about newborn infants in the way we now think about fetuses when we allow a woman to abort a defective fetus and to try again to have a normal child'.

When there is a dispute over the care or rights of a baby, then the courts become involved and that usually means more prolongation of life and presumably of suffering – not only for the child. Cases have become famous, particularly in the USA, where parents have fought lengthy battles with the courts to let their babies die. The case was reported in 1989 where:

> A Chicago man held police and hospital personnel at bay with a pistol while he disconnected his son's life-support system. Fifteen-month-old Samuel Linares had been in coma on a ventilator for several months, showing no sign of recovery. Yet hospital staff were unwilling to stop treating him. After taking Samuel off the ventilator, his father cradled him in his arms as he died (*IME Bulletin,* 1989b).

The father was not indicted for murder.

The case of 'Baby J' was well reported in the press in 1990. He was born at twenty-seven weeks gestation with a birth weight of 1.1 kg. He required ventilation but had times when he could breathe spontaneously, and could also be looked after at home. It took several court decisions not to resuscitate him again when he next came to that point. The Master of the Rolls, on giving judgement, quoted from a Canadian document of a similar case:

> There is a strident cry in America to terminate the lives of other people – deemed physically or mentally defective... Assuredly one test of civilization is its concern with survival of the 'unfittest', a reversal of Darwin's formulation... In this case, the court must decide what its ward would choose,

if he were in a position to make a sound judgement (*IME Bulletin,* 1990a).

The shock that parents experience at the birth of a malformed or handicapped baby is often enough for them either to reject the child, or not be able to make logical decisions. Occasionally, decisions will have to be made fairly rapidly if the baby is to live. Probably more often it is true to say that decisions can wait two or three days, by which time the parents may have had some time or occasion to adjust to the birth, and the condition of the child itself will have given some indication of how well he or she may survive. Nevertheless, a decision will have to be taken.

The ethical dilemma is always, to let live, or to let die.

At birth it is impossible to decide what IQ a child with Down's syndrome may attain. On the other hand, a baby born with spina bifida or other congenital malformations may have a high IQ but be subjected to an existence which may seem intolerable. But is it so to him or her? And life is more than just the IQ. The kind of attention a handicapped infant receives at birth may very well determine his or her future life. Is it not again the quality and depth of the significant relationship which matters, and which may be the most important element in such a dilemma?

At the end of life

As it is far from easy to determine when life begins, so it is not easy to decide when life ends, or should end. The added dimension in the debate, at least for adults, is that the person concerned often feels that she or he would like to have some control over the manner of their dying. With the increasing use of medical technology this is often not easy.

Death has come to be seen as something that, like illness, should not really be there. Death is seen as the culmination of illness, and in a way the worst illness. As most illness is dealt with in hospitals, so death happens in hospitals. This has all meant that death has become something which most people are not familiar with, and which goes on 'out there'. What one does not see as a regular event one is not accustomed to and consequently afraid of.

The social conditions, at least in the western world, have also improved drastically. When 'living' was no more than misery and poverty, death was something desirable, because the after-life promised freedom from all that.

Illnesses and diseases which not so long ago were 'the old man's friend', that is, acceptable as easing the passage from life into death, are now a mere few tablets away and no more than an occasional inconvenience for someone. Living longer means postponing death. The reality of it is still there, but because medicine is able to postpone it again and again, death has become the 'outrage' and that which should not happen.

These are perhaps unspoken generalizations, but much of society's behaviour is in that direction. The accompanying issue is a spiritual one: what one doesn't have to face one forgets about. With a loss of religious values and practices, death has lost its desirability and its mystique. Hence it is feared, and is avoided.

The question 'When does life end?' is equally difficult to answer as 'When does life begin?' Cessation of breathing and heart beat are not clear enough indicators of death.

Brain death has become one of the criteria for establishing death. With artificial ventilation it is possible to keep a person's lungs and heart functioning even though there are no other signs of life such as cranial nerve or reflex functions. There are clear guidelines for establishing brain death, and these have to be followed in cases of doubt or dispute.

One of the reasons for a diagnosis of brain death is the possible use of organs for transplantation. When brain death has been diagnosed, a person may be kept ventilated for some time, usually not more than seventy-two hours, for this purpose.

Some of the ethical dilemmas facing people are around issues of death-care, not of health-care. The same machines which help a baby to live have created the problem of how and when to let someone die.

The right to die

There has been a long debate, particularly in the United States, about a person's right to die. This underlies the debate about euthanasia.

An American court case in June 1990 found it very difficult to uphold a person's right to die (*IME Bulletin,* 1990a). The patient was a young woman who had had a car accident. She was found without detectable respiratory or cardiac function, but paramedics were able to restore breathing and heart beat. After three weeks in a coma she progressed to an unconscious state in which she was able to take nutrition. But after it became apparent that she had virtually no chance of recovery, her parents asked that artificial hydration and nutrition should be discontinued. This was based on her:

> expressed thoughts at age twenty-five in somewhat serious conversation with a housemate friend that if sick or injured she would not wish to continue life unless she could live at least halfway normally [and] that given her present condition she would not wish to continue on with her nutrition and hydration.

The court felt that they could accept a person's right to refuse treatment, but could not accept that her parents were entitled to order the termination of her medical treatment. (There is in the report a reference to 'her then husband' referring to the time shortly after the accident.)

- Can a court of law decide on the 'quality of life' of a person, or can only a medical person decide that?
- Should the parents of an adult rendered incompetent have the right in law to decide on her behalf?

This and an earlier case (see page 139) happened in America, and nothing similar has been reported in Britain. That fact is not conclusive: it *could* happen here as well. The dilemma is that a person, now incompetent, cannot decide about what should happen, and so nobody else can either. The court cannot decide about someone's quality of life, and neither can it accept that the family's feelings are necessarily in the patient's best interest.

The decision, it seems, is not to decide, and that seems to lead to that 'fate worse than death'.

- Have we become the prisoners of our own inventions?

Euthanasia

The World Medical Association issued the following statement about euthanasia in 1987:

> Euthanasia, that is the act of deliberately ending the life of a patient, either at his own request or at the request of his close relatives, is unethical. This does not prevent the physician from respecting the will of a patient to allow the natural process of death to follow its course in the terminal phase of sickness (*IME Bulletin*, 1987b).

A distinction is usually made between different types of euthanasia.

Passive euthanasia

Passive euthanasia, mercy death, or negative euthanasia is taking a direct action for shortening life by withholding helpful treatment *because that person has requested it*. It has also been referred to as assisted suicide.

Active euthanasia

Active euthanasia, mercy killing or positive euthanasia is taking a direct action to terminate a person's life *without that person's permission*.

Voluntary euthanasia

Voluntary euthanasia means that the individual has freely given consent to his death after having been fully informed.

Involuntary euthanasia

Involuntary euthanasia means purposefully shortening someone's life without that person's consent.

None of these are at present legal in Britain, nor in most other countries. However, Holland is usually cited as the country where euthanasia happens openly and regularly. This is probably not correct. The Dutch Supreme Court has laid down guidelines for doctors, and if these have been followed, there is a good chance that the acts of euthanasia will not be prosecuted:

1   The request for euthanasia must come only from the patient, and must be entirely free and voluntary.
2   The patient's request must be well-considered, durable and persistent.
3   The patient must be experiencing intolerable (not necessarily physical) suffering, with no prospect of improvement.
4   Euthanasia must be the last resort. Other alternatives to alleviate the patient's situation must have been considered and found wanting.
5   Euthanasia must be performed by a physician.
6   The physician must consult with an independent physician colleague who has experience in this field (*IME Bulletin*, 1989c).

Most people would agree that to die with dignity is preferable to lingering and suffering. The difficulty is usually, whose values or rights have precedence: the patient's or the doctor's?

At the time of writing the 'living will' forms available in Britain are not legal documents. A person may have written that she or he does not want to have life-saving treatments in certain situations, but a doctor is not bound to respect this. He is, however, bound by his code to preserve life, and that is often the overriding motive.

• Whose life is being respected?

Because of this, many people feel very strongly that they need to look after their own rights, and by various means (e.g. living wills, or 'Advance Declarations' as the Voluntary Euthanasia Society calls them in Britain, and giving power of attorney) ensure that their wishes are respected in situations where they may not be able any more to decide for themselves.

It is significant that in many instances where somebody has helped a dying relative to take some medication, or has not given a prescribed dosage, they have not been judged guilty of killing or murder (*Daily Telegraph*, 1990). The circumstances have usually been considered as mitigating in their favour.

The line between passive euthanasia and pain control can, however, be a very subtle one. Many more nurses are better trained in pain control and palliative care and can, therefore, accept that large doses of diamorphine given correctly are not euthanasia, but in fact good patient care.

The care which patients receive at the end of their lives is perhaps the most contentious of ethical problems for nurses. Nurses often feel that patients are not cared for appropriately – or that doctors prescribe tests and treatments which they consider inappropriate – and that they need to challenge this.

Letting someone die

The opposite of euthanasia must be good care of dying patients.

Allowing people to die is not abandoning them without care. Neither does it mean that someone is thereby not given any chance to choose to live or die. Allowing someone critically ill without hope of recovery to die means, however, to 'accept death' which is part of Thiroux's (1980) principle of the value of life.

Letting someone die is perhaps the most difficult choice for many doctors. On the other hand, many a patient will feel that she is 'ready', or that he has literally had enough, and has no more strength to fight for life. When that is acknowledged and accepted by *all* concerned – patient, relatives and friends, doctors, nurses – then it must surely be right to allow the natural process of dying to take place.

Ordinary and extraordinary means

The terms 'ordinary' and 'extraordinary' have been used 'to insist that it is the patient's ultimate interest which should determine the treatment he receives' (Dunstan, 1981). Ordinary means of preserving life indicate what is normal, established and well-tried, giving a reasonable hope of benefit and causing only acceptable pain, inconvenience or disturbance. Extraordinary means of preserving life, on the other hand, would be treatments, investigations and medications whose immediate or long-term benefits are doubtful, cannot be obtained or used without pain, cause psychological disruption to the patient, and are of disproportionate cost.

Some extraordinary means have become ordinary over time. Dunstan (1981) lists general anaesthesia, analgesia in childbirth and (many) surgical interventions as those which have changed from one to the other already, and organ transplants as being in the transition at present.

What are the choices?

It may sometimes seem, when considering what happens at the end of life, that whichever way one turns it is wrong. We live too long, we die too long. We have technology, but like the sorcerer's apprentice, we seem unable to stop its *destructive* aspects.

Some of the issues described may be brought into focus by a case history:

> Danny was a 23-year-old man who had originally come from the West Indies to study in Britain. He had stayed on doing postgraduate studies. A rather introverted person, Danny had often gone away at weekends on his motorbike. During one such outing he had an accident which left him not severely injured, but unconscious. He recovered from his injuries. He never needed ventilating, and was being fed via a naso-gastric tube.
>
> Time passed, and as he was still unconscious, without family, and had only one or two friends who visited less and less often, the nurses felt he was their special patient. This was evident by the way they cared for him. His situation was reviewed in a case conference after six months and again after a year. Each time the conclusion was to see how events would turn out, but that if any infection set in, he would not be treated. But Danny had no infections, and no sores anywhere. Two years after the accident a case conference was held again and doctors and nurses came to the conclusion that his condition was unlikely to change now. It was decided to withdraw nourishment and to continue with watery liquids only. He eventually died about six weeks later.

This case must be on the borderline between euthanasia and letting die. It is unusual in that there was no other person involved who had any claim on Danny except his health care staff.

The subject of euthanasia is an emotive one because words like killing and murder are used for actions which concentrate only on one side of the problem.

Against this, the care of the elderly leaves still often much to be desired. Those who are also mentally ill can cause tremendous problems. Old, demented, but alive and often very much 'kicking', they are a burden on families and society, and often on themselves.

Even when they can still care for themselves, they have lost their friends, their interests are different from those around them, and they are dependent on those who are good enough to spare them an hour or two. They have to ask and then be grateful for the smallest service. Is it not understandable that many of them wish they could die?

Those who, like Danny and the American woman (see pages 141–2) are in hospitals take up a bed and resources which could be used for someone more acutely ill. The question of economics versus a person's life is often acutely difficult to reconcile (see Chapter 4).

Perhaps it is also that a person's spiritual or transcendent needs and values are being forgotten in this age of technology, and a whole aspect of life and death is overlooked by blindness caused by the shiny stainless steel of life-saving equipment.

This may be the aspect of the debate about euthanasia which has been missing for too long. The relationships a person has with the self, with others, and with God have, on the whole, not been used as equal criteria. In an ethic of caring they are, however, at the centre. The emphasis here is on the relationship between the patient or client and the significant other in his or her life.

It may be possible – and in many instances it is – that just as life could be said to begin when there is a relationship between mother and fetus, so life ends when the relationship between the patient and his or her significant other has ceased. When a person has become unconscious for a long time there comes a point when her husband, friend or whoever is closest, detaches emotionally from her. There is no means of reciprocating their relationship. There is no way in which the patient can any longer 'receive'. The two cannot respond to each other any more. It is often felt as if the patient – the other – is dead already. There is no longer a meaningful relationship. The essence of personhood is response-ability, and without that, the person is no longer a person. 'What criteria have to be fulfilled to call *some-body* a corpse?' asks Wackers (1990). Could it be that the breakdown or breaking up of the significant relationship is one of them?

The person who asks for active euthanasia for another, once-loved person has a heavy responsibility. This is why such a decision is surely never taken lightly. Seeing someone suffer is immensely difficult. Seeing that someone deteriorate, lose dignity and literally be a shadow of his former self is also degrading to the one who watches this with increasing suffering.

On the other hand, the person who asks for euthanasia, or for cessation of treatment, may not so much be asking for *less* treatment as for *more* – but more of a different kind: more attention, more help with facing death – or with living meaningfully, if that is the case. The request for euthanasia both for self and for another, must always be considered also as a cry for help.

By saying that the relationship should be one of the criteria for or against euthanasia, it is clear that someone needs to have insight into that relationship. Someone – perhaps a nurse – needs to be so close to patient and significant person that she or he can discern what that relationship is. That person, that nurse, is one who listens, who hears, responds, advocates, respects, trusts, and above all, cares. That person, out of what she or he hears, will be able to respond in such a way that ethical problems are seen as human problems. Principles of life, good, right, justice, truth and freedom are seen in perspective and applicable to this one unique situation. It may be a question of doing what is right and dutiful, or would be in the best interest of all, but above all it is a question of doing what is creative and healing in this situation, between these people involved here. Then dying and euthanasia become 'human'. Kennedy (1990) complained that 'the real enemy is not death – it is inhumanity'. When humanity is back in it, death also is not an enemy, but more a part of the whole scheme of things.

The 'crucial moral task is to perceive accurately the situation in which one is called upon to act' (Keks, 1984). This is indeed what Niebuhr (see Chapter 2) sees as the outcome when the question 'what is happening?' is answered correctly, responsibly and therefore morally.

This still leaves many practical aspects of euthanasia to consider:

- Who is the most significant person in a relationship and who decides this?

By listening and hearing this will emerge. It may not be the 'obvious' person.

- How can claims of love, and those of economics, be reconciled?

Perhaps when the carer has seen how the relationship works, the answer may emerge.

• When and how should a nurse intervene when she or he believes that a patient is receiving too much inappropriate treatment?

Advocacy is based on the person's (patient's) *needs*, not the nurse's wants or desires.

• How can the care of dying patients be improved so that the care is more ethical, beneficial and human, and less unethical, harmful and inhuman?

By knowing what principles are involved, and being aware of professional responsibilities and carrying them out.

When nurses are dealing with families and friends of dying persons, they can give them support and care. When, as in the case of Danny, the nurses themselves are the significant others, they themselves need support – and a lot of it. Their decision meant literally undoing their own work over the last two years. There will have been many questions to ask in that case, and many to answer, about very many different aspects of their care and relationship, which it would be impossible to mention here. That support may be like an evaluation of nursing altogether, but specific to this case will have been the relationship. And:

> Instead of assessing . . . results or the rules of an ethical code, we . . . can ask, what was the nature of the relationship between the various people involved? [We need to] evaluate the nature of the relationship between those seeking help and those offering help in professional health care. It is here that we most urgently need criteria for moral judgement (Campbell and Higgs, 1982).

Perhaps an ethic of caring is not only an ideal in dilemmas, but a workable tool? Not for giving *the* answer, but a human and creative answer in the unique situation which every person presents.

10

Ethics and the future

Into the future

Ethics will always deal with situations which are on the borderline between the acceptable and the not (yet) acceptable. This is why ethics is so difficult, and so important. What is accepted and acceptable is not disputed. But what is disputed is how the (as yet) unacceptable is to be made acceptable – or not.

Ethics is, therefore, a thing of the moment. Some topics are here today and some tomorrow. By touching on certain topical aspects in ethics in this chapter, it must be evident that in a short time they will not be 'hot' in the same way. Nevertheless, the way in which they are dealt with today will shape how tomorrow's topics will be viewed and dealt with.

In the middle of life

The ethical issues which concern people at the beginning and end of life are different from those which present themselves to people in the middle of their lives. And yet they all hang together: a decision about birth control influences the beginning of life, and embryo research has to do with sanctity of life, and who or what is controlling it, and how long a fertilized embryo can or should live.

The main difference between this part of life and the two earlier ones is that here the individual concerned is more in charge and personally taking the decisions which concern him or her rather than, by and large, having the decisions made about him or her.

Many of the ethical issues here are concerned with sexuality: its expression, its success and its use.

Contraception

Contraception has passed into general practice and the main talking point about it seems to be not *if*, but *which*. Research continues to find better and more reliable methods and medications which are safer and have less potential side-effects.

Contraception is still not officially acceptable for Roman Catholics, though many people of that church practise it. They feel that this is their choice and that they should not be dictated to by the church. Other people feel that it is not possible to follow only the acceptable parts of a church's teaching. In countries where the Roman Catholic church is strong, people usually have large families.

In the West, people tend to consider that contraception is a personal choice. In the East, the opposite is true, and countries like China and India have strong family planning policies. There the opposite is true, and families are exhorted to have only one child.

A decision at one end of the world literally has repercussions at the other end.

Safer sex

Safer sex practices have been widely publicized in recent years to prevent the spread of AIDS. This usually means using some form of contraception.

To practise safer sex means essentially also to restrict oneself to fewer sexual partners – ideally a one-partner relationship. It is difficult to combine the opposing values of fidelity to one partner and sexual freedom because condoms are now liberally available.

- Society seems to be giving a double message; is it adding to the confusion about sexual mores, or shaping them?

Artificial fertilization

The ethical debate around artificial fertilization centres more around the methods: AID (artificial insemination by donor) or AIH (artificial insemination by husband). Which technique is better, or more ethically acceptable? There may be many reasons for choosing either the one or the other method.

It is believed that about one in six couples in the UK will need help to conceive a child (Meerabeau, 1985). For many of these couples *in vitro* fertilization (IVF) or gamete intra-fallopian transfer (GIFT) offer the only chances of having a child. The first 'test-tube baby' made history, but since then there have been hundreds more. Nevertheless, the technique is not yet easy or risk-free, nor even highly successful. Because several eggs have to be harvested, fertilized and implanted, multiple pregnancies are likely, resulting also in many perinatal deaths.

- Is it ethically right and emotionally bearable to produce multiple pregnancies when the babies so born are too small to survive?

In 1986 a report (*IME Bulletin* 1986a) listed sixteen different ways of making artificial insemination possible. The same report also carried an item about the possibility of male pregnancy, adding that to acquire a baby there are still also 'the "old-fashioned" ways possible of normal sexual intercourse and adoption; in some countries one should include also donation, purchase and theft'.

Surrogacy

Surrogacy may be an age-old answer to the age-old problem of childlessness. Recent practices have, however, brought this problem into sharp focus because it has been done for financial gain.

Several countries (among them Australia and the USA) have laws to prohibit surrogacy. The ramifications of surrogate motherhood are many, often resulting in court cases where the surrogate mother is unwilling to give up the child, or the commissioning couple is unable to adopt the child once born. If the child is in any way handicapped or ill this adds yet another dimension.

Embryo research

The Report of the Committee of Enquiry into Human Fertilization and Embryology (*Warnock Report*, 1984) had been commis-
sioned because embryo research had become widely practised
and was beginning to be controversial. It has, however, taken
the government until 1990 to put the Human Fertilization and
Embryology Act onto the statute books. The Human Fertilization
and Embryology Authority is responsible for seeing that the Act
is carried out and adhered to.

Perhaps the main debate in recent years has been on the time-
limit for research on embryos, and to what this research should
be limited. Human embryos can be used for studying both normal
and abnormal human development, and also for cloning – that
is, for asexual reproduction of tissues. They can also be used for
testing drugs. Trans-species fertilization is another area of research
where sperm is used to fertilize hamster eggs to investigate male
infertility. The Act regulates these various practices. The time-
limit of fourteen days was set earlier for research on embryos.
This is the longest time span of any European country; most of
whom allow research on embryos only until five to eight days.

The subject is a fascinating one. It stretches the imagination
into all sorts of possibilities. But its practical implications are as
diverse as its imaginary possibilities.

- Who owns any spare embryos?
- With their potential for life, are they simply 'waste'?
- The genetic information in stored or frozen embryos could
  potentially be used for good or ill – who decides?
- Research on human embryology goes alongside research in
  biology – can the two help each other? For good or ill?
  Research in genetics can be used to combat disease and create
  disease. Where is the line?
- 'Genetic engineering' is an emotive term – what sort of a
  'Brave New World' do we want to create?

Molecular genetics has identified the genes responsible for muscu-
lar dystrophy and cystic fibrosis. Links have also been made
between some psychiatric disorders and genetic factors. Manic

depressive psychosis, schizophrenia and Alzheimer's disease may all be biologically-based disorders, and alcoholism may also have a genetic basis. These findings make it possible that at-risk populations may be tested (Gournay, 1990). This could be a good thing, but again, where is the line drawn between preventing disease and creating a world where only perfectly healthy people have a place?

So far, the only possible way of putting this type of genetic research into practice is in the cases of hereditary diseases. The *in vitro* fertilized ova can be examined at the six or eight cell stage for their sex. Certain types of hereditary diseases, such as Huntingdon's chorea which develop only in males can, therefore, be eliminated in that only female pre-embryos are then transferred to the mother.

This opens the field wide for selecting only desirable 'material' for pregnancy. While it seems reasonable not to subject a child to a life of illness and early death, it seems more questionable when a couple simply wants a boy or a girl to use these techniques to suit their fancy – or to ensure that a certain title can be carried on.

Eugenics, as 'the science which deals with all influences that improve the inborn qualities of a race; also... those influences that develop them to the utmost advantage' (Roberts, 1981) seems to have become a respectable science after the efforts of the Nazis to create the super-race. Without legislation it is, however, perfectly legitimate that atrocities could be perpetrated again.

An ethic of caring does not mean that it is against advances and improvements. An ethic of caring will want to put the human element into the middle of the debate about scientific possibilities:

- What are the needs of the people concerned?
- Does a childless couple feel they are pressured into *in vitro* fertilization because it is 'the done thing'? Has someone heard their deep needs? Is it possible to stand back and ask 'what is happening?'.
- What happens emotionally to children born of IVF? Does the fact that their embryo has been frozen have any psychological effect?
- What about the cost of such programmes? Does it mean that money spent on IVF is not available for other care, perhaps

care of the elderly, handicapped or mentally ill? Does it mean
that our parents are less well cared for than our children?
- Ethical principles of:
  - the value of life
  - goodness and rightness
  - justice
  - truth
  - individual freedom
  are all implicated and have to be considered, not only by the
  people directly involved, but by everyone. These issues *do*
  concern everyone.

An ethic of caring will always ask the questions – and seek the
answers – which concern the people involved. It will ask the
questions which nobody else might have asked, and it will not be
afraid to ask the obvious or simple questions. It will always ask
about feelings, fears and hopes. These are the things which matter
between people.

Organ transplants

The area of organ transplants is never out of the news. The
ethical considerations mostly concern the risks involved in the
procedure, and the unpredictable results. Only corneal grafting
can be done with a high degree of success at present, because it
is a largely avascular procedure.

Most organs or tissues for transplantation are taken from dead
donors. Live donors are used less often because of the obvious
risks of a major operation, and the rejection rate is high. The
incident in 1989 of the sale of kidneys raised this issue into the
limelight.

> This commercial trafficking in living human organs has been
> generally condemned as a horrific exploitation of the poor
> (Evans, 1989).

Government moved swiftly and introduced the Human Organ
Transplants Act in April 1989 which prohibits the sale of human
organs and stipulates that living organ donors be genetically
related to their recipient. This latter can be suspended in
cases which satisfy the Unrelated Live Transplant Regulatory
Authority (ULTRA).

Organ transplants have become a regular part of care for patients. The most widely used organs (after corneas) are kidneys, and heart-and-lung transplants have become commonplace. Perhaps the main difficulty with such procedures nowadays is their procurement. The most common donors are accident victims, and asking their already distraught relatives to consent to organ transplants is not easy. 'The person who approaches possible donor families is often delegated to do so according to position or status rather than because he or she has empathy or the skill to do it well' (Coupe, 1990). Like all skills of communication, this has to be learnt. Asking relatives for organs may mean asking them for a favour when they are already grieving, but it also means that another person can therefore live and this may be a fitting memorial to the deceased.

The other frequent means of obtaining organs is from patients in intensive therapy units who have been diagnosed brain dead. Such patients can be kept ventilated until suitable recipients for their organs are found and prepared. 'This opens a whole new debate about the use of resources and the practice of doing something to a patient that will be of no benefit to him' (Coupe, 1990). This is probably the aspect of organ transplantation which is most difficult and questionable for nurses.

In an ethic of caring the relationship between carer and cared-for is of paramount importance. It is a reciprocal relationship, which means that both parties are equally important. When one of the people involved is not able any longer to respond, then there is more responsibility put on the other. When that other, in this case the nurse, cannot share with the recipient what is happening to her or him, then that sharing has to be done somewhere else. Usually this is seen as support for the nurse. In this particular situation this may mean not just emotional support, but a need for a forum to voice ethical and moral points, and be *heard*. Too often the support offered may be the kind of holding operation until the nurse 'has got over' a difficult time. This may not be enough, because it may be more than the pain of severing a human relationship; the practice of keeping alive may be questioned, and may have to be taken up in settings where it can and will be discussed. The question facing a nurse could indeed be:

- Is it equally unacceptable, from a moral point of view, to treat the dead as if they were living as it is to treat the living as if they were dead? (Wackers, 1990).

This aspect of organ transplants questions more closely than others what life and death are about. Is a transplant a neat way of defying death? It could be argued that the less death is accepted, the more death is in a sense destroying life: more and more scarce resources mean less and less health care for all. Ramsey's (1970) famous phrase of surgeons 'slashing and suturing their way to eternal life' has an uncomfortable ring of truth about it. These aspects are causing distress, and they have to be faced, otherwise nurses in particular will not want to work in intensive therapy units.

But equally another question has to be considered:

- [Are we] approaching a time where a person with multisystem failure will be able to have a new heart, lungs, liver, kidney and legs, a face lift, skin grafts and new eyes – colour of their choosing. Where will it end. How do we control it? Will Frankenstein become a reality? (Satterthwaite, 1990).

It is not possible to divorce organ transplants from these questions. And the neighbouring issue is always that of scarce resources. Even if someone had the money to pay for every replacement available, is it right that it should be done?

A very different type of transplant is that of fetal brain cells for people with Parkinson's disease. This practice was started in 1988 and there were reports of successful outcomes. The implications of such practices can again be very widespread. Research has to be carried out on fetuses to make such procedures feasible, and the possibility of women having abortions for gain could be envisaged.

The situation has arisen a few times where a pregnant woman has been maintained on a life support system, although brain dead, until the fetus she was carrying can be safely delivered by Caesarean section. Although in the cases reported (*IME Bulletin*, 1986b) the children were normal neurologically, the possibility of later emotional difficulties must surely exist.

Most contributions to the debate about transplants concentrate on the donor, and the medical and ethical issues concerned with that. Few mention the recipient, and the impact a transplant might have on him or her. Yet we usually associate the heart with emotions of love, the kidneys with consciousness and emotions of fear, the brain with personality and memory. Looked at physiologically, these organs are not carriers of emotions, but if these organs were not seen to be linked with the person as a person, then what makes a person unique?

An ethic of caring does not dismiss these issues. Indeed, because a transplanted organ means that a very special kind of relationship is being formed with a person – unknown, and now dead – who has given something of himself or herself, this surely must have some impact on the recipient?

- Is there a biological integrity which is being breached when an organ is exchanged?
- What feelings does a person have after a life-saving operation when an organ was transplanted?
- What about the people who don't want to accept a transplant for deep moral reasons?
- Is it right to want to continue with kidney dialysis (which is more expensive) even when a kidney would be available (thus saving money)?

Transplants have become a way of life; 'spare-part surgery' is now commonplace. But the way organs are obtained still causes anxiety. When technology and simple person-to-person communication, i.e. relationships, have learnt to go hand-in-hand, then perhaps other anxieties around the subject will die away.

As above, in this area too, Utopian ideas are being considered very seriously. Cryonics – deep-freezing the body for possible reanimation many years hence – is beginning to be a financial proposition. In 1990 there were apparently fifteen British and about 120 American people subscribing to a scheme, with thirteen people currently already 'suspended' in the USA (Edghill, 1990). At this stage there must surely be an anxiety about what would happen if there were a power-cut....

Ethics committees

With so many areas of research and new practices it is obvious that some control is necessary. Some, like embryo research, is nationally controlled. But individuals may carry out research which also reaches to the limits of acceptable practice. This may be trying out a new operation, or a new combination of drugs. It may also be the questioning of a particular patient group about certain behaviour or styles of living which may not appear to have any connection with the disease, or trying different methods or treatment and comparing them with patients in control groups.

Many hospitals and health authorities have had ethics committees for a long time, but on the whole they are more often non-existent, or where they do exist, seldom if ever meet. The general trend is quite clearly for ethics committees to exist and function effectively in more and more places.

Such committees should examine clearly any requests for research in their area. This may be submitted by doctors, nurses, or any other health care personnel in their authority.

In the past any such ethics committees were largely made up of physicians, surgeons, clergymen and perhaps one lay person. Increasingly it is seen that lay persons need to have a larger input, and that nurse representation is essential. Nurses and lay persons in particular play a vital role in often defending the interests of the patients and not simply letting a request pass 'on the nod' because the doctors present approve it. They do not always know better, and such a committee is important if decisions are to be impartial and not seen as supporting the interests of its members.

To sit on ethics committees is a new experience for many nurses. Their own research has tended not to be controversial and needing the approval of an ethics committee. But this is changing and nursing research now increasingly reaches into areas where approval is necessary. This means that nurses on such committees also gain greater insight into preparing such research; not rigorous enough preparation simply means that a project could be rejected which might have been very worthwhile. (The IME has a 'Standard application form for ethical approval of research proposals'. Available from: IME Office, 13/14 Great Sutton Street, London EC1V 0BX, Telephone 071 608 0842.)

These practices highlight, particularly for nurses, the importance of informed consent, and of advocacy and also accountability. The need for such committees is illustrated by the following story:

Fiona was a staff nurse, just qualified, on a children's ward. She had overheard the registrar saying something about research to a colleague a few days earlier but had thought nothing about it. Then she noticed that two of the young children, due for operation the next day, both had premedications written up in dosages which were large even for adults. She checked with the sister who did not seem alarmed; as the registrar had written the prescription, 'he must know what he is doing'. Fiona checked with the pharmacy, who were horrified. They in turn checked with the manufacturer, who gave clear guidelines for the dosage for children. Fiona became suspicious, remembering the remark about research. She phoned the hospital administrator to find out if there was an ethics committee in the hospital, and was told no. She finally got hold of the registrar to check the dosage with him. He assured her it was correct. She then told him of her investigations, and asked him which ethics committee had sanctioned the research and whether or not the parents had consented to it? He appeared on the ward quickly to change the dosage to that recommended for children of that age.

Many people – not only doctors – still feel that they can try a good idea on some unsuspecting patient and get away with it. This is nothing short of deception and contrary to every rule in every code which stresses trust and respect. Kant's best-known phrase must surely be to 'treat humanity, whether in your own person or in that of another, always as an end and never as a mere means'. This is not a bad motto for any ethics committee.

There has been talk for some time of a national ethics committee but at present this has not happened yet. The Royal College of Nursing has an ethics committee which has an advisory function and meets when called upon to discuss a particular point or situation.

Ethics in Europe

The European Community is no longer a novelty but a fact, and increasingly there will be more cooperation not only between businesses and industry, but also between health care personnel.

It may be useful to take a brief look at the bioethics scene in Europe. The following information is all taken from the monthly

IME Bulletins. (The number in brackets following an item refers to the *IME Bulletin* Number from which the information came.)

France

Doctors in Lyons performed a feto–fetal cell transplant. The baby was diagnosed antenatally to be suffering from a rare immune deficiency. Cells were taken from the liver and thymus of two aborted fetuses and injected into the umbilical cord of the affected fetus. At seven months old, the child had had no serious problems. (49)

In December 1982 a law was passed to define the conditions under which research on human subjects may lawfully be carried out. The law also established a network of regional multidisciplinary committees to protect research subjects. (51)

A Life Sciences and Human Rights Bill was stalled early in 1990, possibly fatally. This Bill would have allowed research on embryos up to seven days, with the National Ethics Committee able to grant extensions to fourteen days. (55)

Denmark

The Danish Council of Ethics is required by law to advise the Minister of Health on legislation on embryo research, embryo storage, genetic diagnosis of embryos, and various other aspects of assisted procreation. (51)

Norway

In June 1989 the Norwegian parliament established three national research ethics committees with a brief for medicine (health and life sciences), normative academic disciplines and natural science/technology. (51)

Germany

Following a television programme in January 1989, German medical schools withdrew slides and specimens which were used for teaching purposes and contained material from bodies of concentration camp victims. (48)

The West German government is having great difficulty in

passing an Embryo Protection Bill. (60)

The unification of East and West Germany in October 1990 has highlighted the different abortion laws in the two parts. The number of abortions carried out in both countries is about equal in number, but West Germany has a population about 3.5 times larger than East Germany. After unification the differing laws will continue for two years side-by-side, but without punishment.

In 1989 there were a number of protests in Germany against a speaker at a European Symposium on 'Bioengineeri g, ethics and mental disability'. The speaker was to give a paper entitled 'Do severely disabled newborn infants have a right to life?' Attacks were also made on other lecturers. (The two speakers most attacked were Drs Kuhse and Singer, cited on page 138.) It seems that the subject of euthanasia is taboo in Germany because of what happened during the Nazi era, when euthanasia was equated with a power which the doctors would have, and that they are not to be trusted with any such powers because of the role they had in Hitler's regime. The development of racial purity, with its consequences of forced sterilization and involuntary euthanasia, has since become a subject which can simply not be discussed. (61)

Austria

Similar protests also took place in Austria in 1990 where a lecture about euthanasia had to be cancelled. Handicapped people had protested that human life is inviolable. (63)

Italy

The membership of the Italian national bioethics committee had to balance many competing political interests, and therefore consists of forty members of various disciplines – rather more than in most other countries.

Poland

Poland used to have a fairly liberal abortion law but since democratization the Roman Catholic church's influence has increased to the point where abortion is almost completely prohibited. (62)

Romania

Romanian children with AIDS have been much in the news. It has become clear how this happened: blood was not screened for HIV, and giving blood secured favours, which was useful for homosexuals who were outlawed. Hospitals were set up to keep very sick babies alive in order to avoid formal investigations on the death of an infant under one year old. Small blood transfusions of 50–100 ml were given to malnourished children, with the well-known results. (64)

USSR, Czechoslovakia, Bulgaria

In these countries there is no teaching of medical ethics to medical students, although in Bulgaria some subjects are covered in teaching by the Institute of Social Medicine. (52)

European legislation

There is increasing legislation on ethical matters concerning the member states of the European Community.

In October 1989 the Council of Europe adopted a statement on Ethical Issues of HIV Infection in the Health Care and Social Settings. (58)

In March 1990 the Council published recommendations concerning medical research on human beings. (56)

In July 1990 the Directorate-General of the European Commission published Guidelines on Good Clinical Practice for Trials on Medicinal Products in the European Community. These guidelines came into operation on 1 July 1991 and will probably be turned into a directive in 1992. (64)

In December 1989 there was a proposal put forward for a European ethics committee as 'a place where scientists, lawyers, politicians and "wise men" could share ideas'. (57)

This overview is very piecemeal and mostly directed at doctors, and 'wise *men*'. There is little mention of nurses and wise *women* here: this could be seen more as an opportunity than just an omission. The invitation to put an ethic of caring into the middle of any debate, local, national and international, is wide open.

Postscript

Someone once said that if ethics is taught properly, standards of care will never have to be taught. This seems a remarkably good piece of advice. The only difficulty is, that it is very hard to teach ethics properly. It seems to be all clear, and then another area comes into view and another aspect opens up which was not thought about.

An ethic of caring is in a way combining these two aspects: ethics and standards of care. Essentially it is about people, patients and nurses (specifically) or health care personnel. When they relate to each other and talk and listen *with* each other, then ethics happens, and the standard of care is at its highest.

Ethics is about social justice, equality and respect, and education is the basis of that. Caring is about loving – not romantic love, but the kind of love St Augustine meant when he wrote 'Love, and do what you want'. When love is truly there, then there is no question that what is done is right. Perhaps the various ways of expressing profound truths all come to the same thing, and that can also be said as 'Love your neighbour as yourself' or 'I and Thou'.

The essence lies not in saying these things, but in *doing* them, and in *being* truly there, truly present.

References

Allbrecht T. (1982). What job stress means for the staff nurse. *Nursing Administration Quarterly*, **7** (1), pp. 1–11.

Anonymous (1988). Research without consent continues in the UK. *Institute of Medical Ethics Bulletin*, **40**, pp. 13–15.

Anonymous (1989). Editorial. *Nursing Times*, **85** (21), p. 3.

Aroskar M. A. (1980a). Anatomy of an ethical dilemma: the theory, the practice. *American Journal of Nursing*, **80** (4), pp. 658–63.

Aroskar M. A. (1980b). Ethics of nurse–patient relationships. *Nurse Educator*, **5** (2), pp. 18–20.

Bailey R. (1985). *Coping with Stress in Caring*. Oxford: Blackwell

Baly M. (1984). *Professional Responsibility* (2nd edn). Chichester: Wiley.

Benjamin M. and Curtis J. (1986). *Ethics in Nursing* (2nd edn). New York: Oxford University Press.

Bergman R. (1976). Evolving ethical concepts for nursing. *International Nursing Review*, **23** (4), Issue 208, pp. 116–17.

Binnie A. et al (1984). *A Systematic Approach to Nursing Care*. Milton Keynes: Open University Press.

Bond M. (1986). *Stress and Self-awareness: A Guide for Nurses*. Oxford: Heinemann.

Broad C. D. (1930). *Five Types of Ethical Theory*. London: Routledge and Kegan Paul.

Brown M. (1985). Matter of commitment. *Nursing Times*, **81** (18), pp. 26–7.

Brown P. (1986). Who needs an advocate? *Nursing Times*, **82** (32), p. 72.

Buber M. (1937). *I and Thou*. Edinburgh: T and T Clark Ltd, Translation (1970) by W. Kaufman.

Campbell A. V. (1984a). *Moderated Love*. London: SPCK.

Campbell A. V. (1984b). *Moral Dilemmas in Medicine* (3rd edn). Edinburgh: Churchill Livingstone.

Campbell A. V. and Higgs R. (1982). *In That Case*. London: Darton, Longman and Todd.

Candee D. and Puka B. (1984). An analytic approach to resolving problems in medical ethics. *Journal of Medical Ethics*, **10** (2), pp. 61–70.

Carlisle D. (1989). The hell called Leros. *Nursing Times*, **85** (39), p. 18.

Carr A. (1985). Professionalism, curse or blessing? *Lampada*, **3**, pp. 42–5.

Churchill L. (1977). Ethical issues of a profession in transition. *American Journal of Nursing*, **77** (5), pp. 873–5.

Committee of Enquiry into Human Fertilisation and Embryology. *Warnock Report* (1984). London: HMSO.

Coupe D. (1990). Donation dilemmas. *Nursing Times*, **86** (27), pp. 34–6.

Cox C. (1979). Who cares? Nursing and sociology: The development of a symbiotic relationship. *Journal of Advanced Nursing*, **4**, pp. 237–52.

Crabbe G. (1988). The lonely dilemma. *Nursing Times*, **84** (9), p. 18.

Cupitt, D. (1990). The value of life. *The Modern Churchman*, **XXXII** (2), pp. 39–45.

Curtin L. L. (1979). The nurse as advocate: a philosophical foundation for nursing. *Advances in Nursing Science*, **1** (3), pp. 1–10.

Daily Telegraph (1990). News: Judge frees pair who tried to kill dying mother, 14 November.

Davis A. J. and Aroskar M. A. (1983). *Ethical Dilemmas and Nursing Practice*. Norwalk, Conn: Appleton-Century-Crofts.

Downe S. (1990). Conflict of interests. *Nursing Times*, **86** (47), p. 14.

Duncan A. S., Dunstan G. R. and Welbourne R. B. (1981). *Dictionary of Medical Ethics* (2nd edn). London: Darton, Longman and Todd.

Dunstan G. R. (1981). Life, prolongation of: Ordinary and extraordinary means. In *Dictionary of Medical Ethics* (2nd edn)

(Duncan A. S., Dunstan G. R. and Welbourne R. B., eds.). London: Darton, Longman and Todd.

Edel A. (1955). *Ethical Judgment*. Glencoe, New York: The Free Press.

Edghill S. (1990). Living past your sell-by date. *Ms London*, 26 November, p. 20.

Edwards T. H. (ed) (1984). *Living Apocalypse*. London: Harper and Row.

Egan G. and Cowan R. M. (1979). *People and Systems: An Integrative Approach to Human Development*. Belmont, Cal: Brooks/Cole.

Eliot T. S. (1944). *Four Quartets*. London: Faber and Faber.

Epting S. (1981). Coping with stress through peer support. *Topics in Clinical Nursing*, **2** (4), pp. 47–59.

Eriksson K. (1976). Nursing – skilled work or a profession? *International Nursing Review*, **23** (4), Issue 208, pp. 118–20.

Evans M. (1989). Kidneys for sale: the real evil. *IME Bulletin*, **48**, pp. 13–15, March.

Faulder C. (1985). *Whose Body Is It?* London: Virago Press.

Flanagan L. (1986). A question of ethics. *Nursing Times*, **82** (35), pp. 39–41.

Ford N. M. (1988). *When Did I Begin?* Cambridge: Cambridge University Press.

Fox M. (1979). *A Spirituality Named Compassion*. Minnesota: Winston Press.

Frank A. (1958). *Anne Frank's Diary*. London: Valentine, Mitchell and Co Ltd.

Frankl V. (1962). *Man's Search for Meaning*. New York: Pocket Books.

Gaze H. (1985). The unequal equation. *Nursing Times*, **81** (7), pp. 16–17.

Gillon R. (1986). *Philosophical Medical Ethics*. Chichester: Wiley.

Gournay K. (1990). A return to the medical model? *Nursing Times*, **86** (40), pp. 46–7.

Gramelspacher G. P. et al (1986). Perceptions of ethical problems by nurses and doctors. *Archives of Internal Medicine*, **146**, pp. 577–8. In *IME Bulletin*, **13**, p. 4.

Handy C. (1983). *Taking Stock*. London: BBC.

Häring B. (1978). *Free and Faithful in Christ* (Vol. 1). Slough: St Paul Publications.

Harris J. (1987). QALYfying the value of life. *Journal of Medical Ethics*, **13** (3), pp. 117–23.

Havard J. (1985). Medical confidence. *Journal of Medical Ethics*, **11** (1), pp. 8–11.

Henderson V. (1966). *The Nature of Nursing*. New York: Macmillan.

Heywood Jones I. (1988). The buck stops here. *Nursing Times*, **84** (17), pp. 50–2.

Heywood Jones I. (1989). Condoning ill-treatment. *Nursing Times*, **85** (43), pp. 39–40.

Higgs R. (1985). Case conference: A father says 'Don't tell my son the truth'. *Journal of Medical Ethics*, **11** (3), pp. 153–8.

Hodges C. (1990). Value for money? *Nursing Times*, **86** (14), p. 20.

Horan F. and Jackson V. (1984). Abortion: who decides? *Nursing Times*, **80** (10), pp. 16–18.

Illich I. (1976). *Limits to Medicine*. Harmondsworth: Pelican.

International Council of Nurses (1973). *Code of Nursing Ethics*. Geneva: ICN.

IME Bulletin (1986a). News and notes: Male pregnancy, **14**, pp. 12–13, May.

IME Bulletin (1986b). News and notes: Life after death, **17**, p. 15, August.

IME Bulletin (1987a). Law report: Sterilisation of mentally retarded girl is authorised, **26**, pp. 7–9, May.

IME Bulletin (1987b). News and notes, **31**, p. 13, October.

IME Bulletin (1989a). Review: When does human life begin?, **46**, pp. 13–17, January.

IME Bulletin (1989b). News: Infant not murdered, **50**, p. 6, May.

IME Bulletin (1989c). News: Euthanasia in Holland, **53**, p. 8, September/October.

IME Bulletin (1990a). Law report: US Supreme Court defends right to die, **60**, pp. 23–4, August.

IME Bulletin (1990b). Law report: Court permits doctors not to resuscitate gravely handicapped infant, **63**, pp. 22–3, November.

Jameton A. (1984). *Nursing Practice: the Ethical Issues*. Englewood Cliffs, NJ: Prentice-Hall.

Johnston W. (1981). *The Mirror Mind*. London: Collins.

Jourard S. M. (1971). *The Transparent Self*. New York: Van Nostrand Reinhold Co Inc.

Kalisch B. J. (1971). Strategies for developing nurse empathy. *Nursing Outlook*, **19** (11), pp. 714–17.

Keighley, T. (1986). Accountability. *Nursing Standard*, (**466**), 2 October.

Keks J. (1984). Moral sensitivity. In *Ending Lives* (Campbell R. and Collinson D., eds (1988)). Oxford: Blackwell.

Kennedy L. (1990). *Euthanasia: the Good Death*. London: Chatto and Windus.

Kratz C. (1984). Minorities and power. *Lampada*, **1**, pp. 41, 43–5.

Kuhse H. and Singer P. (1985). Handicapped babies: A right to life? *Nursing Mirror*, **160** (8), pp. 17–20.

Langford M. (1985). *The Good and the True*. London: SCM Press.

Lawrence J. and Crisham P. (1984). Making a choice. *Nursing Times*, **80** (29), pp. 57–58.

Liss P-E. and Nordenfelt L. (1990). Health care need, values and change: How changed values influence an evaluistive concept. In *Changing Values in Medical and Health Care Decision Making* (Jensen U. J. and Mooney G. eds) Chichester: Wiley.

Lyall J. (1989). A human reaction. *Nursing Times*, **85** (38) p. 19.

Lyall J. (1990). Cycles of evasion. *Nursing Times*, **86** (34) pp. 16–17.

McCarthy D. (1986). Blowing the whistle. *Nursing Times*, **82** (11), pp. 31–3.

MacDougall R. H., Orr J. A., Kerr G. R. et al (1990). Fast neutron treatment for squamous cell carcinoma of the head and neck: final report of the Edinburgh randomised trial. *British Medical Journal*, **301** (6763), pp. 1241–2.

MacIntyre A. (1985). *After Virtue* (2nd edn). London: Duckworth.

Mahoney J. (1984). *Bioethics and Belief*. London: Sheed and Ward.

May W. F. (1975). *Code, Covenant, Contract or Philanthropy*. Hastings Center Report 5, December, pp. 29–38.

Mayeroff M. (1972). *On Caring*. New York: Harper and Row.

Meerabeau L. (1985). Infertility under the microscope. *Nursing Times*, **81** (17), p. 20.

Melia K. (1984). Cracking the new code. *Nursing Times*, **80** (43), p. 20.

Mill J. S. (1967). *Utilitarianism*. London: Longmans.

Mitchell T. (1984). Is nursing any business of doctors? *Nursing Times*, **80** (19), pp. 28–32.

Moore D. (1988). Confidentiality: all sewn up? *Senior Nurse*, **8** (6), pp. 6–7.

Niblett W. R. (1963). *Moral Education in a Changing Society*. London: Faber and Faber.

Niebuhr H. R. (1963). *The Responsible Self*. New York: Harper and Row.

Noddings N. (1984). *Caring – a Feminine Approach to Ethics and Moral Education*. Berekeley, CA: University of California Press.

Nouwen H. J. M. (1987). Out of solitude. In *The Human Act of Caring* (Roach M. S., ed.). Ottawa: Canadian Hospital Association.

Nouwen H. J. M. with McNeill D. P. and Morrison D. A. (1982). *Compassion*. London: Darton, Longman and Todd.

Nursing Times (1983). News, **79** (26), 29 June.

Nursing Times (1985a). News, **81** (9), 27 February.

Nursing Times (1985b). News, **81** (19), 8 May.

Nursing Times (1986). News, **82** (24), p. 6, 11 June.

Nursing Times (1987). News, **83** (37), p. 10, 16 September.

Nursing Times (1988). News, **84** (50), p. 6, 14 December.

Nursing Times (1989). News, **85** (21), p. 7, 24 May.

Oakley, A. (1984). The importance of being a nurse. *Nursing Times*, **80** (50), pp. 24–7.

Partridge K. B. (1978). Nursing values in a changing society. *Nursing Outlook*, **26** (6), pp. 356–60.

Pearson A. (1983). *The Clinical Nursing Unit*. Oxford: Heinemann.

Porter S. (1988). Siding with the system. *Nursing Times*, **84** (14), pp. 30–1.

Ramsey P. (1970). *The Patient as Person*. New Haven: Yale University Press.

Rankin-Box D. F. (1988). *Complementary Health Therapies: a guide for nurses*. Beckenham: Croom Helm Ltd.

Raths L. E., Harmin M. and Simon S. (1966). *Values and Teaching*. Columbus, Ohio: C. E. Merrill.

RCN (1980). *Guidelines on Confidentiality in Nursing*. London, RCN.

Rea K. (1985). Dishonouring the code. *Nursing Times*, **81** (2), p. 17.

Roach M. S. (1985). *Caring as Responsibility: A Response to Value as the Important-in-itself*. Paper delivered at 2nd International Congress on Nursing Law and Ethics, Tel Aviv, June.

Roach M. S. (1987). *The Human Act of Caring*. Ottawa: Canadian Hospital Association.

Roberts D. F. (1981). Eugenics. In *Dictionary of Medical Ethics* (2nd edn) (Duncan A. S., Dunstan G. R. and Welbourne R. B., eds). London: Darton, Longman and Todd.

Rogers C. (1961). *On Becoming a Person*. London: Constable.

Rogers C. (1978). *On Personal Power*. London: Constable.

Sacks J. (1990). Reith Lectures: 2 The Demoralisation of Discourse. *The Listener*, **124** (3192), pp. 9–11.

Sale D. (1990). *Quality Assurance*. Basingstoke: Macmillan.

Salvage J. (1985). *The Politics of Nursing*. Oxford: Heinemann.

Salvage J. (1990). The theory and practice of the 'new nursing'. *Nursing Times*, Occasional Paper, **86** (1), pp. 42–5.

Satterthwaite H. J. (1990). When right and wrong are a matter of opinion. *Professional Nurse*, **5** (8), pp. 434–7.

Saxton D. F. and Hyland P. A. (1979). *Planning and Implementing Nursing Intervention* (2nd edn). St Louis: C.V. Mosby.

Scott R. S. (1985). When it isn't life or death. *American Journal of Nursing*, **85** (1), pp. 19–20.

Seedhouse D. (1988). *Ethics: The Heart of Health Care*. Chichester: Wiley.

Sieghart P. (1985). Professions as the conscience of society. *Journal of Medical Ethics*, **11** (3), pp. 117–22.

Sigman P. (1979). Ethical choice in nursing. *Advances in Nursing Science*, **1** (3), pp. 37–52.

Simmons D. (1982). *Personal Valuing: An Introduction*. Chicago: Nelson Hall, pp. 98–101.

Steele S. M. and Harmon V. M. (1983). *Values Clarification in Nursing* (2nd edn). Norwalk, Conn: Appleton-Century-Crofts.

Stewart K. and Rai G. (1989). A matter of life and death. *Nursing Times*, **85** (35), pp. 27–9.

Stover E. and Nightingale E. O. (1985). *The Breaking of Bodies and Minds*. Oxford: W. H. Freeman and Co Ltd.

Swaffield L. (1990a). Euro-diseases. *Nursing Times*, **86** (34), p. 42.

Swaffield L. (1990b). System failures? *Nursing Times*, **86** (23), p. 21.

Thiroux J. P. (1980). *Ethics, Theory and Practice* (2nd edn), Encino, Cal: Glencoe Publishing Co Inc.

Thomason C. (1987). *Advocacy and the Development of Community Care*. Discussion Paper 547, Personal Social Services Research Unit, University of Canterbury.

Thompson I. A., Melia K. and Boyd K. (1983). *Nursing Ethics*. Edinburgh: Churchill Livingstone.

Thornton S. (1984). Stress in the neonatal intensive care unit. *Nursing Times*, **80** (5), pp. 35–7.

Tingle J. (1990a). When to tell. *Nursing Times*, **86** (35), pp. 58–9.

Tingle J. (1990b). Ethics in practice. *Nursing Times*, **86** (48), pp. 54–5.

Trevelyan J. (1988). Agents of repression. *Nursing Times*, **84** (42), pp. 45–7.

Tschudin, V. (1991). *Beginning with Awareness.* (A training package.) Edinburgh: Churchill Livingstone.

Tschudin V. with Schober J. (1990). *Managing Yourself.* Basingstoke: Macmillan.

Turner T. (1989). Taking the lead. *Nursing Times,* **85** (43), pp. 16–17.

Turner T. (1990a). Crushed by the system? *Nursing Times,* **86** (49), p. 19.

Turner T. (1990b). Moral imperatives. *Nursing Times,* **86** (39), p. 19.

UKCC (1984). *Code of Professional Conduct.* London: UKCC.

UKCC (1985). *Advertising by Registered Nurses, Midwives and Health Visitors.* London: UKCC.

UKCC (1986). *Administration of Medicines.* London: UKCC.

UKCC (1987). *Confidentiality: an Elaboration of Clause 9 of the Second Edition of the UKCC's Code of Professional Conduct.* London: UKCC.

UKCC (1989). *Exercising Accountability.* London: UKCC.

Wackers G. L. (1990). Building networks: A constructive perspective on changes in medicine and health care. In *Changing Values in Medical and Health Care Decision Making* (Jensen U. J. and Mooney G., eds). Chichester: Wiley

Walsh P. (1985). Speaking up for the patient. *Nursing Times,* **81** (18), pp. 24–7.

Way H. (1962). *Ethics for Nurses,* Nursing Times publication.

Weale A. (ed) (1988). *Cost and Choice in Health Care.* London: King Edward's Hospital Fund for London.

Webb C. (1987). Speaking up for advocacy. *Nursing Times,* **83** (34), pp. 33–5.

White C. (1985). Jack – a study in anguish. *Nursing Times,* **81** (41), pp. 24–6

Wolfsenberger W. (1977). A multi-component advocacy protection scheme. In *Advocacy and the Development of Community Care.* (Thomason C., ed (1987)). Discussion Paper 547, Personal Social Services Research Unit, University of Canterbury.

Yeager J. (1977). Why I had to strike. *American Journal of Nursing,* **77** (5), p. 874.

Index

Abortion, 53, 117, 133–7
  in Europe, 162
Abuse, 124
Accountability, 71, 103,
  110–16, 129, 159
'Advance Declaration', 144
Advertising, 70–1
Advocacy, 97–100, 108, 118,
  129, 149, 159
Aloneness, 14
Altruism, 74, 128
Answerer, 62
Artificial fertilization, 152,
  154–5
Assault, 124
Assertiveness, 25–6
Assessment:
  of problem, 85–7, 105,
    118, 135
Attitudes, 29, 30–1
Autonomy, 61
  nursing, 101–2, 111, 125,
    129

Babies, malformed, 138
'Baby J', 139–40
Becoming, 38
Being, 37
Beliefs, 28–9
Beneficence:
  principle of, 60
Brain death, 141, 156

Capital punishment, 53
Care-giver, nurse as, 9–12
Care-receiver, concept of,
  12–13, 15
Caring, 1–16
  components of, 1–9, 14
  duty to, 76
  models of, 17–27
  purpose of, 47
  relationship, 13–16, 147
  response ethics and, 61–3
  role of nurses, 27
  standards of, 110
  uniqueness of, 1, 44
  values of, 35–9
Case notes, confidentiality of,
  94–6
Challenging medical opinion or
  treatment, 104–9, 117–21
Children:
  confidentiality and, 24–5
  consent of, 21
Choices, 82–3
Citizen, 62
Clarity, 37
Code(s), 18–19, 64–71, 81
  confidence in, 7
Coercion, 116
Colleagues, ethical issues
  between, 122–4
Collegial model, 18
Commitment, 8–9, 14, 36, 45,
  89, 119, 138

Communication, 38
  confidentiality and, 24–5
  values of, 44–5
Community, 25, 63
Companionship, 15, 45
Compassion, 4–6, 14, 36, 47,
  119, 138
Competence, 6, 14, 36, 68,
  115, 119, 138
  competitiveness and, 5
  extra duties and, 75
  of patients, 21
Complementary therapies, 126
Conduct, professional, 86
Confidence, 7, 14, 36, 101,
  119, 138
Confidentiality, 24–5, 94–6
Conflicting claims, 24–5, 116,
  121
Conscience, 7–8, 11, 14, 36,
  119, 138
Consent, informed, 19–22, 159
Consequentialism, *see*
  Teleology
Contraception, 151
Contract, 19, 75
  models, 18, 19–22
Cooperation, 117
Courage, 3
Covenant models, 18, 19, 27
Creative(ness), 16
  decision-making, 89–90
  responsibility, 62–3
  values, 29–30
Creativity, 15–16, 55, 88–9,
  129, 135
Crime, confidentiality and, 95
Cryonics, 158

Death, 140–9
  organ transplantation
    following, 156–7
Deception, 23–4, 59
Decision-making, 82–92
  independent, 102–4

Declarations, 71–3
Deontology, 50–1
Descriptive ethics, 47–8
Dialysis, 56
Dilemmas, 131
Duties, 76–7, 80–1, 136
  extra, 75, 114–16

Economy, 41–3, 54
Effectiveness, 41–3
Efficiency, 41–3
Embryo research, 132–3,
  153–5
  in Europe, 161
Empathy, 9–12, 38, 97
Employers:
  nurses and, 109–21
  rights and duties of, 77–8
Engineering model, 18
Equality, 164
Ethic of caring, 85, 87, 89, 92,
  97, 104, 131, 154, 164
Ethics committees, 158–60
  in Europe, 161, 162
Ethics, principles of, 51–61
  theories of, 46–7
Eugenics, 154
European Community, 160–3
Euthanasia, 53, 142–9
  in Germany, 162
Evaluation, 38, 91
  of ethical problems, 91–2,
    107, 120, 137
Experiencing, 30
Experiential values, 30
Extra duties, 75, 114–16

Fairness, principle of, 56–7
Fetal brain cell transplantation,
  157
Five Cs, 3, 14
Freedom, 14, 38
  principle of individual,
    59–60, 61, 119, 135
  to act, 111

Good, concept of, 49
Goodness, principle of, 54,
  119, 135, 155

Handicapped babies, 138–40
Harm, doing no, 55, 60–1, 88
Health, values of, 39–41
Health services, values of, 41–3
Honesty, 2, 30
  principle of, 57–9, 61
Hope, 3
Human rights abuses, 72–3,
  121
Humility, 3

Imperative, practical, 51
Implementation, of problem,
  90, 107, 120, 137
Inclusion, 14
Individual, responding to, 87
Institution, rights and duties of,
  77–8
Integrity, 59, 88
International Council of Nurses
  (ICN):
  Code for Nurses, 64–6
  resolutions, 72–3
In-vitro fertilization, 154

Job satisfaction, 10
Judgement, use of, 112, 116
Judging, 13
Justice, principle of, 56–7, 77,
  119, 135, 155
  social, 164

Knowledge, 2
  informed consent and,
    20–1

Law:
  accountability and, 111
  confidentiality and, 94–6
  consent and, 21–2
  European, 163
  euthanasia and, 143–4

Letting die, 145
Life:
  beginning of, 132–3
  end of, 140–1
  value of, 52–4
Listening, 11, 25, 97, 101, 148
'Living will', 144
Loyalties, 122, 124

Maker, 62
Malformed babies, 138–40
Malpractice, 124
Managers, conflict with,
  116–17
Market forces, 41–3
Meaning, 25, 35, 44, 89, 119
Means:
  ordinary, 145
  extraordinary, 145
Medical opinion or treatment:
  challenging of, 104–9,
    117–21
Misconduct, 122–4
Moral rules, 50–1
Morality, 46

Needs, perceived, 40
'New nursing', 25–7
Nonconsequentialism, *see*
  Deontology
Non-maleficence, principle of,
  60–1, 77, 119
Normative ethics, 47–51
Nuremberg Code, 19–20
Nursing process, 83

Objection:
  conscientious, 121
  to treatments, 117
Obligations, 21, 136
Organ transplants, 155–8

Partnership, 25–7
Paternalism, 22–3, 31, 80, 89
Patience, 2
Patient's Bill of Rights, 78–80

Philanthropy, 22
Planning: in decision-making, 87–90, 106, 119, 136
Policies, 77
Political action, 125–6
PREPP (Post-Registration Education and Practice Project), 124
Priestly model, 17, 22
Principles, ethical, 51–61, 86, 128
Profession, nursing, 124–30
Professionalism, 128–30
Punishment, 23–4, 121

QALY (Quality Adjusted Life Year) theory, 54
Qualpacs, 110

Receptivity, 14, 25, 35, 44
Reciprocity of care, 11
Relatedness, 14, 25, 36, 44
Relationship:
caring, 13, 97, 131, 156
fostering, 119
models of, 17
nursing, 100, 103
professional, 86, 109, 124
trusting, 7
Research:
embryo, 132–3, 153–5
trials, 20, 121
Respect, 37, 109, 164
for the person, 51, 61, 119
Responding to needs, 11
Response ethics, 61–3
Responsibility, 61, 67, 74–5, 80–1, 107, 113, 115, 118, 147
accountability and, 113–14, 117
theory of, 61–3
Responsiveness, 14
Responsivity, 25, 36, 44
Resuscitation, 108
Right, concept of, 49, 50, 54–6

Rightness, principle of, 54–6
Rights, 75–6, 80
of institution, 77–8
of patient, 78–81
to die, 141–2
to life, 138

Safe sex, 151
Self-assessment, 11
Self-awareness, 9–12
Self-defence, killing in, 53
Separateness, 14, 37–8
'Spare-part surgery', 158
Staff shortages, 42, 43
Standards of care, 110
Strike action, 126–8
Suffering, 9, 15
meaning of, 47
'Suffering-in', 9–12
Suicide, 53–4
assisted, 143
Surrogacy, 152

Teleology, 49–50
Theories, ethical, 48–51, 61–3
Torture, 121
Transplantation, organ, 155–8
Treatment, challenging of, 104–9, 117–21
Trust, 2, 7
Truth-telling, principle of, 57–9, 61, 88, 119, 135, 155

United Kingdom Central Council (UKCC):
advisory documents, 70–1
Code of Professional Conduct, 6, 66–7, 68–70, 75, 81, 115, 124, 127
Utilitarianism, 49–50

Value(s), 25, 28–31
attitudinal, 30
of caring, 35–9
creative, 29

examples of, 32–4
experiential, 30
of health, 39–41, 118
of health care, 41–3
moral, 136
of nursing, 43–5, 129
principle of life, 35, 52–4,
    61, 119, 135, 155
questioning of, 31
Value-judgements, 13

Value-statements, 32
Verbal communication, 2, 38
Virtues, 39

War, 53
'Warnock Report', 132
Work conditions, 76, 125
World Medical Association, 72,
    142–3